CONTENTS

Chapter One: Overview

Chapter Two: Adolescent Health Issues

Introduction

Young People and Health is the one hundred and twenty-third volume in the **Issues** series. The aim of this series is to offer up-to-date information about important issues in our world.

Young People and Health provides an overview of the issues involved in adolescent health, including mental health, sexual health, substance misuse, diet and nutrition and self-harm and suicide, before looking at some of these issues in more detail in the second chapter.

The information comes from a wide variety of sources and includes:
Government reports and statistics
Newspaper reports and features
Magazine articles and surveys
Website material
Literature from lobby groups
and charitable organisations.

It is hoped that, as you read about the many aspects of the issues explored in this book, you will critically evaluate the information presented. It is important that you decide whether you are being presented with facts or opinions. Does the writer give a biased or an unbiased report? If an opinion is being expressed, do you agree with the writer?

Young People and Health offers a useful starting-point for those who need convenient access to information about the many issues involved. However, it is only a starting-point. Following each article is a URL to the relevant organisation's website, which you may wish to visit for further information.

*****

Young People and Health

ISSUES

Volume 123

Series Editor

Craig Donnellan

Assistant Editor

Lisa Firth

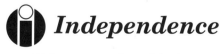

Independence

Educational Publishers
Cambridge

First published by Independence
PO Box 295
Cambridge CB1 3XP
England

British Library Cataloguing in Publication Data
Young People and Health – (Issues Series)
I. Donnellan, Craig II. Series
613'.0433

ISBN 1 86168 362 6

Printed in Great Britain
MWL Print Group Ltd

Layout by
Lisa Firth

Cover
The illustration on the front cover is by
Don Hatcher.

Young people into 2006

A unique contemporary archive of young people, this new report provides the answers to over 100 health-related behaviour questions

Annually since 1986, the Schools Health Education Unit (SHEU) has published the collected Health Related Behaviour Questionnaire (HRBQ) results. Data from more than 700,000 pupils between the ages of eight and 18, have now been recorded since the questionnaire's launch in 1977. More than 5,600 separate school surveys have been carried out, some schools repeating surveys of their pupils on five occasions. The data banks at SHEU are a unique resource that are consulted by a wide range of groups and individuals including local education authorities, public health authorities, government offices, university departments, schools, teachers and other interested individuals.

The 20th report, *Young People into 2006*, shows figures and graphs from youngsters between the ages of 10 and 15. They tell us about what they do at home, at school, and with their friends. The data have been collected from 310 primary and secondary schools across the United Kingdom. The original sample of 37,932 was finally reduced to 17,743 to be much more representative of the country as a whole.

Food choices and weight control

Breakfast
30% of the 14 to 15-year-old females and 22% of the 14 to 15-year-old males had nothing at all to eat for breakfast 'this' morning. (p.2)

Lunch
21% of the 14 to 15-year-old females ate no lunch on their previous day at school. (p.3)

Breakfast and Lunch
36% of the 14 to 15-year-old females who had nothing to eat at breakfast 'this' morning (on the morning of the survey) had nothing to eat at lunch the previous day at school. (p.3).

Healthy eating
Females are more likely than males to take health into account when choosing what to eat. 24% of the 14 to 15-year-old males say they 'never' consider their health when choosing what to eat. (p.12)

Weight
56% of 14 to 15-year-old females and 55% of the 12 to 13-year-old females 'would like to lose weight'. The proportion of the 14 to 15-year-old females who missed breakfast and lunch and 'would like to lose weight' is around 25%. 21% of older males and 15% of older females were 'overweight' using height/weight data. (pp.4 and 7).

Food choices
(The following comments apply to dietary items consumed 'on most days'.) More than 58% of older pupils have dairy products. Females from 10 to 15 years show a greater preference for fresh fruit, salads and vegetables. Data since 1987 reveal a slight downward trend in those choosing crisps and in 2005 35% of 14 to 15-year-olds eat crisps 'on most days'. (pp.8-11)

Legal and illegal drugs

Experience of alcohol
Up to 8% of 10 to 11-year-olds, up to 24% of the 12 to 13-year-olds, and up to 41% of the 14 to 15-year-olds had consumed at least one of the listed alcoholic drinks during the previous week. (p.53)

Beer or lager
24% of the males and 11% of the females, aged 14 to 15, drank at least one pint of beer or lager during the previous week. Figures suggest that fewer are drinking but 'drinkers' are drinking more. (p.56)

Wines and spirits
24% of the 14 to 15-year-old females drank at least one small bottle of pre-mixed spirit drinks during the previous week. 19% of the 14 to 15-year-old females had drunk at least one glass of wine during the previous week. Since 1996, the data shows that older females 'overtook' the males as spirit drinkers and in 2005, 19% of 14 to 15-year-old females reported drinking one or more spirit measures in the past week. (pp.58, 59 and 61)

Alcohol units
17% of 14 to 15-year-old males drank more than 10 units of alcohol 'in the

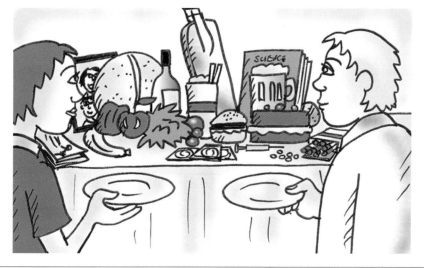

previous week' and 9% of 14 to 15-year-old males drank on three days or more 'last week'. (pp.62-63)

Obtaining alcohol

The off-licence remains the most important source of purchased alcohol, especially for the 14 to 15-year-olds, followed by the supermarket. (p.64)

Drinking at home

Most 'drinkers' drank at home and substantial numbers of 14 to 15-year-olds used other venues including friends, disco, club, party, pubs and outside in a public place. Of those who do drink at home, up to 40% do so with their parents always knowing about it. (pp.65-66)

Smoking levels

24% of the 14 to 15-year-old females and 14% of the 14 to 15-year-old males smoked at least one cigarette during the previous week. 13% of the older female smokers report smoking up to 25 cigarettes a week. (p.67)

24% of the 14 to 15-year-old females and 14% of the 14 to 15-year-old males smoked at least one cigarette during the previous week

---

Sources of cigarettes

15% of the 14 to 15-year-old females were able to buy cigarettes from a shop and 8% of the same group were supplied by friends. (p.68)

Attitude to smoking

Between 12 and 13 years and 14 and 15 years the number of regular smokers triples. Up to 63% will have smoked by the time they are 14 years old. The majority of current smokers say they would like to stop.

Smoking contacts

55% of the older females have a close friend who smokes. The contrast in smoking between females with or without friends who smoke is dramatic, but the highest proportion of all is among females with a 'smoking sister'. Up to 52% of all pupils live in a 'smoky' home. (pp.69-71)

Drug safety

The older they get, pupils think that drugs are 'always unsafe', except

cannabis, which is considered to be 'always unsafe' by a smaller percentage of the older groups. (p.72)

Drug users

Up to 57% of the 14 to 15-year-olds are 'fairly sure' or 'certain' that they know a drug user. (p.73)

Drug experience

About one in five pupils in Year 10 – four times as many as in Year 8 – have tried at least one drug. Cannabis is by far the most likely drug to have been tried, with up to 24% of 14 to 15-year-olds, and up to 6% of 12 to 13-year-olds reporting having taken it. Up to 17% of 14 to 15-year-olds have mixed drugs and alcohol 'on the same occasion'. (pp.74-76)

Exercise and sport

Enjoyment of sport

50% of the 10 to 11-year-old females enjoy physical activity 'a lot'. However, far fewer females than males in each year group report liking sport 'a lot'. Nearly half as many 14 to 15-year-old females as males say they enjoy physical activity 'a lot'. Nevertheless, over 82% of 10 to 11-year-olds and over 64% of the secondary pupils enjoy physical activity 'quite a lot' or 'a lot'. (p.90)

Active sports

Nearly all of the 36 activities listed show a decline in involvement with increasing age except for five-a-side football (males), fitness exercises, golf (males), basketball (males and some females), soccer (males), weight training (males) and 'going for walks' (females). 'Going for walks' is a popular activity for females (up to 38% of older females). Comparing the 14 to 15-year-old 'no active sport' data since 1992 shows a range of 13%-23%. (pp.91-94)

Fitness

Up to 64% of 10 to 11-year-old pupils think they are 'fit' or 'very fit'. 27% of the 14 to 15-year-old females describe themselves as 'unfit' or 'very unfit'. Perceived fitness declines with age in males and females. From 1991 to 2005 there is an upward trend (from 10% to 22%) of 14 to 15-year-old females that report being unfit. (p.95)

Aerobic exercise

Over 85% of all groups (10 to 15-year-olds) had exercised to the level

of 'breathing hard' at least once in the previous week. The gap is seen to widen between males and females among the frequent exercisers as they get older. Up to 14% report never taking exercise in the past week that caused them to breathe harder and faster. (p.96)

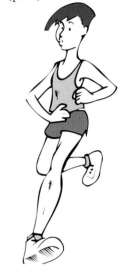

Social and personal

Meeting people of their own age for the first time

Up to 29% are 'quite' or 'very uneasy' (p.99).

Information about sex

Between 12 and 15 years of age there is a trend away from parents and school lessons and a trend towards friends. Parents and/or school lessons should be the main source of information about sex according to these young people. (pp.100-101)

Useful school lessons in health education

Most lessons on the list are reported to be less 'useful' as pupils get older. (p.102)

Enjoyable school lessons

Up to 36% report enjoying 'all' or 'most' school lessons. (p.103)

GCSEs

53% of 14 to 15-year-olds expect good grades at GCSEs (in England, in recent years, around 55% of pupils have achieved grades A to C). (p.104)

After Year 11

60% of 14 to 15-year-old females and 46% of 14 to 15-year-old males want to continue with full-time education. (p.105)

Worries

Around 33% of 10 to 11-year-olds worry about 'family problems'. 14

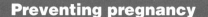

Preventing pregnancy

Year 10 pupils have a choice of four answers to describe best what they know about the list of contraceptive methods. The answers are 'Never heard of it', 'Know nothing about it', 'Not reliable to stop pregnancy', and 'Reliable to stop pregnancy'. Reponses shown in the graph are from the last answer.

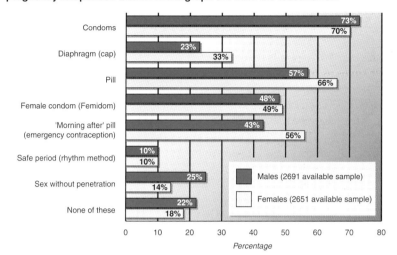

	Males	Females
Condoms	73%	70%
Diaphragm (cap)	23%	33%
Pill	57%	66%
Female condom (Femidom)	48%	49%
'Morning after' pill (emergency contraception)	43%	56%
Safe period (rhythm method)	10%	10%
Sex without penetration	25%	14%
None of these	22%	18%

Males (2691 available sample)
Females (2651 available sample)

Percentage

Source: 'Young People into 2006', SHEU.

to 15-year-old females top the list of most problem areas. 'The way you look' and 'exams and tests' are the principal worries for older females, and 'exams and tests' worry 53% of 10 to 11-year-old females. 50% of 14 to 15-year-old females are worried about the way they look (p.106). Data from *Trends – Young People and Emotional Health and Well-Being 1983-2001* show that since the early 1990s fewer young people report worrying about 'the way you look'.

Schoolwork problems
31% of 14 to 15-year-old females report worrying about schoolwork problems. Up to 26% of all pupils look to the teacher for support. (p.107)

Money problems
25% of 14 to 15-year-old females report money problems and up to 47% of all pupils would talk to their mother and father. (p.108)

Health problems
28% of 10 to 11-year-old females report worrying about health problems and most pupils would turn to their mother and father for support. (p.109)

Career problems
Mothers and fathers are the most likely source of support and the school teacher plays a stronger part for older pupils. 13% of older females would turn to their teacher. (p.110)

Friend problems
Gender differences are pronounced. More males say mother and father,

and 24% of 14 to 15-year-old males would 'would keep it to myself'. More females say mother but up to 34% of older pupils would share the problem with another friend. (p.111)

Family problems
Up to 36% of 10 to 11-year-olds and 38% of 14 to 15-year-old females worry about 'family problems'. Females are twice as likely than males to turn to a friend to share the problem. Males are more likely to go to mother and father and up to 25% of older males would 'keep it to myself'. (p.112)

Bullying problems
15% of 12 to 13-year-old females report worrying about this problem and 21% of 10 to 11-year-old females would share a bullying problem with a teacher. 29% of 14 to 15-year-old males would keep to themselves any problems they experienced with bullying. (p.113)

Self-esteem
The level of self-esteem tends to increase with age. The 'high' group included more males than females. (p.114)

Control over health
The majority feel they are in control of their health. At least a quarter do not think they can influence their health by their own efforts. (pp.115-117)

Getting on with adults
Up to 60% 'get on best' with both parents. Older pupils show a move

away from parents towards other individual family members and friend. Around 75% trust at least two adults. Around 5% of pupils trust no one. (pp.118-119)

Life satisfaction
Males are more satisfied than females. This difference is in line with evidence (p.106) that females worry about more things than males. (p.120)

Sexually-transmitted diseases
In 2003 we reported on the apparent decline in 12 to 15-year-olds' anxiety about the dangers of HIV/AIDS. In 2005 seven to 12% think that HIV/AIDS can be treated and cured. (p.121)

Methods of contraception
Up to 73% selected 'condoms' and up to 66% chose 'The Pill' as the most reliable contraceptive method to stop pregnancy. (p.122)

Methods of contraception reliable to stop infections like HIV/AIDS
Up to 61% chose 'condoms' although there were differences between age and gender e.g. 37% (males) and 39% (females) in the 12 to 13-year-old group compared with 53% (males) and 61% (females) in the 14 to 15-year-old group. (p.123)

Birth control services
56% of the 14 to 15-year-old females knew about a local service for young people, and knowledge grew with age. 49% of the older males did not know of a source of free condoms compared with 36% of the older females. (pp.124-125)

■ The above information is re-printed with kind permission from the Schools Health Education Unit. Visit www.sheu.org.uk for more information.

© SHEU

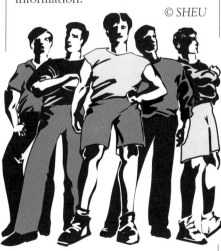

Student health issues

Campus life? It's infectious. Barbara Lantin examines some of the contagious illnesses to which undergraduates are particularly susceptible, and explains how they can best be avoided

Take thousands of students from all over the world, mix them together for the first time, add late nights, too much alcohol and an abysmal diet, and it is not surprising that the outcome is often a trip to the doctor.

'Freshers' flu' is now a recognised phenomenon – the consequence of a sudden, sustained battering to the immune system.

'If you don't eat well, socialise to the early hours on a regular basis and poison your system with alcohol and other recreational drugs, the body will not repair itself so well'

'The student population is at a relatively good time of life in terms of health, strength and vitality,' says Jim Cole, assistant director of the Occupational Safety, Health and Environment Unit at Cardiff University, which runs a student health centre on the campus. 'But if you don't eat well, socialise to the early hours on a regular basis and poison your system with alcohol and other recreational drugs, the body will not repair itself so well.

'Also, students have moved away from home, where they have acquired some immunity to the bugs around them, and into accommodation shared with people from all over the country and abroad, where they will come into contact with a new pool of potential infections.'

A bout of illness in the first year at university is almost inevitable.

A healthy diet, rest and sensible drinking may sound boring, but they are not nearly as tedious as being in bed ill while your friends are out having a great time.

Freshers' flu
What is it and how do you get it?
Just like conventional flu, it is a disease of the lungs and upper airways, caused by the flu virus. This is usually spread in small droplets of saliva coughed or sneezed into the atmosphere by an infected person, or by direct contact with hands contaminated with the virus.
How do you avoid it?
Flu vaccination is recommended only for vulnerable groups, and most students are not in that category. Reduce your risk by not allowing yourself to become too run down. Some people swear that vitamin C, zinc and echinacea prevent them from getting colds; the evidence is mixed.
Symptoms
Fever, shivering, headache, blocked nose, sneezing and a dry cough.
Treatment
Go to bed, rest and drink plenty of fluids. Do not fight it. Take paracetamol to bring down your temperature.

Mumps
What is it and how do you get it?
Mumps is a viral infection of the parotid salivary glands, just below and in front of the ears. The virus is transmitted in the same way as flu and symptoms usually appear two or three weeks after contact. One in four men will get an inflammation of the testes (orchitis) which occasionally leads to infertility.

Cases of mumps multiplied 18-fold in the first third of this year, compared with the same period in 2004, and in the 12 months to July this year there were more than 55,000 suspected cases, compared with fewer than 6,000 the previous year. Universities were particularly badly hit because many people aged 16 to 24 received only one MMR vaccine and two are needed for full immunisation. Earlier this year, health officials warned that up to a third of new undergraduates would not be immunised against mumps and should have a further jab.

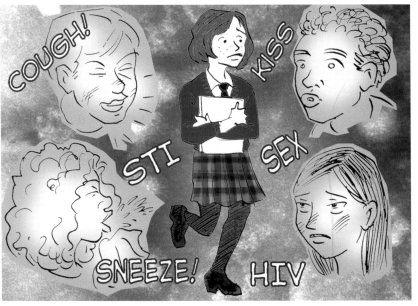

John Addison, 20, a third-year geography student at Keble College, Oxford, began to feel unwell last November after visiting his brother in Cambridge, where mumps was raging. 'By the middle of the week my glands were up and my jaw was stiff. I had a bad headache and felt shattered. The next morning I felt really viral and my cheeks were swollen.

'My mum, who is a nurse, thought it was mumps and the doctor agreed. I'd had the MMR vaccine, so perhaps it wasn't as severe as it might have been. I didn't look ridiculous, but I felt pretty terrible.'

'Students can come into contact with new pools of potential infections'

'It was a bit soul-destroying being in my room at Oxford because nobody could come and see me, so I went home. It was about 10 days before my appetite came back and I felt less tired.'

How do you avoid it?
The MMR vaccine can be given at any age in two doses. Anybody who gets mumps at university should return home as it is highly contagious from a week before symptoms appear to a fortnight after.

Symptoms
The infected glands swell for up to a week, which can make chewing and swallowing painful. Other symptoms include headache, sore throat, tiredness and loss of appetite.

Treatment
Drink plenty of cool fluids, especially water, but avoid fruit juice because it stimulates saliva production, which can be painful. Try holding a warm flannel against the swollen glands. Take a mild painkiller to reduce pain and fever. Men with orchitis may be prescribed a stronger painkiller or corticosteroids.

Meningitis
What is it and how do you get it?
After small children, young adults are most at risk of meningitis, an infection of the membranes that cover the brain and spinal cord. Viral meningitis is more common, but generally less serious. Bacterial meningitis is more dangerous. Both kinds are spread by close prolonged contact, coughing, sneezing and kissing.

How do you avoid it?
Everyone in the UK under 25 should receive the meningitis C vaccine. This does not protect against meningitis B, the most common meningococcal infection. Anyone in close contact with a meningitis patient should visit a doctor.

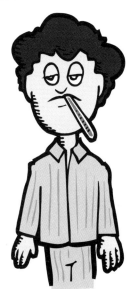

Symptoms
These can be similar to flu and include a severe headache, high temperature, aversion to bright light and an inability to touch the chin to the chest because of neck stiffness. A rash that does not disappear when the skin is pressed with a clear glass is a sign of septicaemia, which can occur in the later stages of meningitis. If the patient's condition is rapidly deteriorating, do not wait for a rash to appear.

Treatment
Meningitis requires immediate hospital treatment, which includes administering antibiotics.

Glandular fever
What is it and how do you get it?
Glandular fever is an infectious illness caused by the Epstein-Barr virus. It is spread in the saliva, and is sometimes known as the 'kissing disease'.

Symptoms
The illness affects the lymph nodes in the neck, armpits, groin and other parts of the body, which can become enlarged. Other symptoms include fever, a very sore throat, inflamed tonsils, exhaustion, muscle aches, a swollen spleen and loss of appetite.

Treatment
There is no cure and the treatment is similar to that for flu. The illness usually runs its course within a month. Avoid vigorous exercise for two months afterwards to protect the spleen.

Sexually-transmitted infections (STIs)
What are they and how do you get them?
There are many STIs, all transmitted by unprotected intimate sexual contact, from genital herpes to HIV. In the nine years to 2004, reported cases of chlamydia, the most commonly diagnosed infection, rose three-fold to more than 30,000 annually and the disease is now thought to affect about 10 per cent of young men and women. In the same time, gonorrhoea rates doubled.

How do you avoid them?
Melissa Dear of the fpa (formerly the Family Planning Association) says: 'Using a condom correctly and consistently when you have sex will prevent the transmission of most STIs, including HIV.' Have regular check-ups at a sexual health clinic: if you notice any unusual symptoms, stop having sex and tell your partner.

Symptoms
One in two men and more than two in three women have no symptoms from chlamydia. Common symptoms of an STI include an unusual discharge, pain or burning on urinating, itches, rashes, pain or bleeding during or after sex and pain in the lower abdomen.

Treatment
Most STIs are treated with antibiotics. If untreated, chlamydia and gonorrhoea can spread to other reproductive organs, causing serious health problems such as pelvic inflammatory disease, ectopic pregnancy or infertility.

7 September 2005

Nutrition through life: teenagers

Information from the British Nutrition Foundation

Key points

- Growth and development are rapid during teenage years, and the demand for energy and most nutrients is relatively high.
- National data shows that average intakes of fat among teenagers were close to the adult benchmark of 35% of food energy.
- A proportion of teenagers had low intakes of some vitamins and minerals (e.g. vitamin A, riboflavin, iron and magnesium), with more girls aged 11 to 18 having low intakes compared to boys of a similar age.
- Teenagers in Britain are largely inactive, with 46% of boys and 69% of girls aged 15 to 18 spending less than the recommended one hour a day participating in activities of moderate intensity.

Energy and nutrient requirements

Growth and development are rapid during teenage years, and the demand for energy and most nutrients is relatively high. This demand differs between boys and girls: boys need more protein and energy than girls due to their greater growth spurt.

The growth spurt usually begins around the age of 10 years in girls and 12 years in boys. In both sexes, an average of 23cm is added to height and 20 to 26kg to weight. Before adolescence, both girls and boys have an average of 15% body fat. During adolescence this increases to about 20% in girls and decreases to about 10% in boys.

One way to obtain sufficient energy (and nutrients) is by the consumption of nutritious snacks to complement regular meals. However, some teenagers eat more than they need and may become overweight, especially if they are inactive. It is better to try to prevent obesity than to encourage strict dieting in this age group. Encouraging a healthy lifestyle is therefore of prime importance during these years. Good habits practised now will be likely to benefit their health for the rest of their lives.

Growth and development are rapid during teenage years, and the demand for energy and most nutrients is relatively high

---

There is an increasing tendency for teenagers, particularly girls, to control their weight by unsuitable methods such as smoking or adopting very low energy diets. A recent government survey reporting on the diets of British schoolchildren found that one in six girls aged 15 to 18 years were dieting to lose weight. A restricted diet, especially one that excludes whole food groups, can lead to nutrient deficiencies and problems in later life.

During adolescence iron requirements increase to help with growth and muscle development. After menstruation begins, girls need more iron than boys to replace menstrual losses. It is difficult to estimate the number of teenagers who are anaemic but the National Diet and Nutrition Survey of young people published in 2000 found that 1% of boys aged 15 to 18 had a haemoglobin level lower than the limit for men and 9% of girls had a haemoglobin level lower than the limit for women. The survey also found many teenage girls had a low intake of iron, with 45% of 11 to 14-year-olds and 50% of 15 to 18-year

-olds having intakes below the lower reference nutrient intake (LRNI), implying that their intakes were likely to be inadequate. Those who start a poorly-planned vegetarian diet or are slimming may be particularly at risk. Bread flour is fortified with iron by law and iron is also added to most breakfast cereals. This makes breakfast an important way of acquiring iron. Although many adolescents do not eat breakfast, these foods can be encouraged as snacks instead together with food or drink containing vitamin C, e.g. citrus fruit or a glass of fruit juice to enhance the absorption of iron.

The rapid increase in bone mass in teenagers means that they require more calcium than adults. Boys should aim for 1000mg per day and girls for 800mg. Good sources of calcium include dairy products (such as milk, yogurt and cheese). Low fat milk and dairy products contain at least as much calcium as whole milk and its products. If these are not eaten, a calcium-fortified soya drink can be a useful substitute. In the UK, white and brown flour (but not wholemeal, which already has an adequate amount) must be

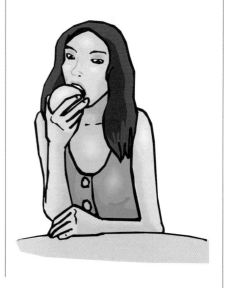

fortified with calcium, so bread made from these flours is a significant source of calcium for many people. Pulses, nuts, dried fruit and green vegetables, such as spring greens and broccoli, contain calcium. But it is a myth that spinach is a good source of minerals – although they are present they are closely bound to digested substances in the spinach, which prevents their absorption. Fish that is eaten with the bones, such as whitebait or canned sardines, are also a good source. In some areas of the country, hard water provides a significant amount of calcium. An additional source of calcium is calcium-rich mineral water.

Current intakes

The National Diet and Nutrition Survey of young people, published in 2000, found the following.

- The main sources of dietary energy were cereal and cereal products, including bread, biscuits, buns, cakes and pastries, which together provided a third of dietary energy. Other sources of energy in the diet included vegetables, potatoes and savoury snacks, which together contributed 15% of energy in boys and 19% in girls, and meat and meat products, which provided 15% of energy in boys and 13% in girls.
- Both sexes exceeded the recommendation that only 11% of food energy to come from non-milk extrinsic sugars (NMES), with boys and girls aged 11 to 18 consuming on average about 16% of energy from NMES.
- Boys aged 15 to 18 consumed more coffee, tea and carbonated drinks than younger boys.
- Girls aged 15 to 18 also consumed more tea and coffee than younger girls as well as more rice, vegetable dishes, bottled water and wine.
- Average intakes of fat were close to the adult benchmark of 35% of food energy. Currently there is no specific benchmark for children's intake of fat, although the adult value is considered relevant for school age children.
- Average intakes of saturates were higher than the adult recommendations (14% vs 11% of food energy).

- Some children had low intakes of some nutrients, with more girls aged 11 to 18 having vit-amin and mineral intakes below the LRNI compared to boys of a similar age. Intakes below the LRNI are likely to be inadequate.
- Excluding salt added during cooking and at the table, daily sodium intakes were already higher than the reference nutri-ent intake (RNI). The mean intake was 2.7g in boys aged 11 to 14 years; 3.3g in boys aged 15 to 18 years; 2.3g in girls aged 11 to 14 years and 2.3g in girls aged 15 to 18 years. This equates to 6.75g, 8.25g, 5.75g and 5.75g of salt, respectively. Average target salt intakes for population groups in children are 5g/day for children aged 7 to 14 years and 6g per day for those aged 15 and over.

Teenagers need a varied diet, incorporating all the major food groups. In the short-term this will help with general appearance (e.g. shiny hair and healthy skin) and energy levels, while in the long term it will help prevent diseases such as cardiovascular disease and osteoporosis.

Physical activity

National data suggest that a majority of teenagers in Britain are largely inactive, with 46% of boys and 69% of girls aged 15 to 18 spending less than one hour a day participating in activities of moderate intensity. The 2004 report *At Least Five a Week, Evidence on the impact of physical activity and its relationship to health* from the Chief Medical Officer recommended that teenagers (and children) have at least 60 minutes of at least moderate intensity exercise every day. It also recommended that activities that increase muscle strength and flexibility and also improve bone strength should be included at least twice a week.

Eating disorders

Anorexia nervosa, bulimia nervosa, binge eating disorders and their variants are psychological illnesses characterised by a serious disturbance in eating, as well as distress or excessive concern about body

shape or weight. Eating disorders are typically seen in girls and young women, but increasingly in teenage boys. Anorexia nervosa is the refusal to eat enough to maintain a normal body weight. Sufferers are of the impression that they are overweight and often picture themselves as being fat even though they are underweight. In teenage girls (and women), anorexia may lead to menstrual abnormalities including cessation of periods, which may have a serious effect on bone health.

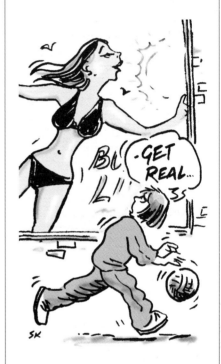

Bulimia nervosa sufferers are also obsessed with the fear of gaining weight. There is a recurring pattern of binge eating, which may be followed by self-induced vomiting. People with bulimia often have an overconcern with their body weight and shape and may feel a lack of control. The foods eaten tend to be high in carbohydrate and fat. Sufferers may also use large quantities of laxatives, slimming pills or strenuous exercise to control their weight. Many bulimics have poor teeth due to regular vomiting. Vomit is acidic and can erode teeth.

- The above information is re-printed with kind permission from the British Nutrition Foundation. Visit www.nutrition.org.uk for more information.

© *British Nutrition Foundation*

Addictions: the basics

Smoking, alcohol, drugs and even gambling are all potentially highly addictive. But you probably already knew that

Why not take a look at how some of these addictions can affect your life. At least you'll be in the know.

Smoking

Young people sometimes start smoking out of curiosity, because they feel that holding a cigarette makes them look older, peer pressure or because it makes them feel like they belong. This is despite the fact that cigarettes are jam packed full of poisons (even the low tar or 'light' brands) which can cause all kinds of fatal diseases.

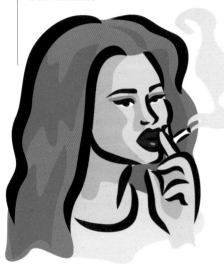

An estimated 450 young people take up smoking each day, and as a sign of how addictive smoking can be, research has found that 70 per cent of adult smokers originally started smoking between the ages of 11 and 15 years old.

But around 120,000 people die from smoking-related diseases each year, many more than the 3,500 that die in road accidents each year, as well as costing you a fortune – a 20-a-day smoker will spend over £1,500 a year on cigarettes.

It's not easy to quit smoking, but there is plenty of help available. Research proves that the longer you smoke, the more you wish to give up and it becomes more difficult to do so.

Alcohol

More than 90 per cent of adults in Britain drink alcohol and a large proportion of young people do too. People drink for a variety of different reasons – to socialise with friends, with a meal in a restaurant, or to help them relax.

But alcohol misuse can be harmful, and young people are especially at risk when drinking because the effects of alcohol can vary dramatically depending on a person's size and weight, along with the type of alcohol they are consuming.

Drugs

Whether you are thinking about using drugs yourself or know someone else who is using them – it's a good idea to know the facts.

Some drugs are more dangerous than others. Class A drugs, including heroin, cocaine, crack, LSD and ecstasy are the most dangerous. These drugs are highly addictive and can cause serious problems with anxiety, paranoia, heart problems or convulsions. You can also die from an overdose.

Gases, glues and aerosols can cause instant death the first time they are tried. Drugs such as cannabis also affect coordination, increasing the risks of accidents, especially if driving.

Drugs are also highly illegal. For example, if you are caught with a Class A drug such as ecstasy you could get up to seven years in custody. If you are under 18 you could be sent to a youth offender's institution or another form of secure accommodation. Supplying someone else with ecstasy (including just sharing drugs) can get you life imprisonment and an unlimited fine.

Class B drugs, like speed, are also illegal. In January 2004, cannabis was reclassified from a Class B drug to a Class C drug. The purpose of this was to make it clear that experts knew that cannabis was harmful, but not as harmful as other Class B substances. Despite the change, it's still illegal to grow, possess or supply cannabis to another person. The maximum penalty for supplying and dealing in cannabis will stay at 14 years imprisonment.

If you want to know more about drugs and their effects, or if you are worried about a friend or relative who may be using drugs, Talk to Frank via the free, confidential drugs information and advice line on 0800 776600 (open 24 hours a day) or visit the Talk to Frank site (www.talktofrank.com).

Gambling

For many gamblers, picking a winning horse or winning the jackpot on a gambling machine can be a real thrill.

But gambling can get out of hand. It is possible to become so addicted to the thrill of winning that gamblers find they start spending more and more time and money trying to win. People with a gambling problem can sometimes find themselves at the mercy of a vicious circle.

Like alcohol or drugs, gambling can be an addiction where the sufferer finds it impossible to live without a bet. Problem gamblers will resort to increasingly desperate measures to fund their habit, including stealing from family and friends. Many addicts find they are unable to pay for food or accommodation.

If you're concerned that your gambling habit has become a problem and would like to speak to someone about it, take a look at the useful links on the Need2Know site.

■ The above information is reprinted with kind permission from Need2Know. Visit www.need2know.co.uk for more information.

© Crown copyright

Adolescent mental health

Study paints bleak picture of adolescent mental health

A huge number of young people suffer from mental health problems that adversely affect their lives, according to research published yesterday by The Priory.

The study by a group of adolescent mental health experts depicts a society in which young people are experimenting with sex, drugs and alcohol, dealing with violence in relationships and at home, and contemplating suicide at an ever-younger age.

Their research is based on interviews with 1,000 young people in England as well as analysis of figures from the Office for National Statistics.

It found that more than one million adolescents have wanted to self-harm, and more than 800,000 have done so. Nearly one million young people have felt so miserable that they have considered suicide, with more than one in five 18 to 19-year-old girls admitting to feeling this way.

Dylan Griffiths, a psychiatrist at the Priory Ticehurst House Hospital, said that 30 years ago it was rare to see young people who self-harmed. 'Today, self-harming is a dramatic, addictive behaviour, a maladaptive way for growing numbers of youngsters to relieve their psychological distress by literally cutting themselves off from disturbing thoughts and feelings,' he said.

Half a million young people had experienced bullying or violence at home, and the same number felt troubled because they weren't sure of their sexuality.

When it comes to alcohol and drugs, the study found 'marijuana, cocaine and alcohol are as ubiquitous as traffic on the street for today's teens'. Nearly five million 12 to 19-year-olds admitted to drinking alcohol, including 49% of all 13-year-olds. Nearly two and a half million young people had been offered illegal drugs, and almost two million had used them.

Marjorie Wallace, chief executive of the mental health charity Sane, said the calls it received from young people reflected The Priory's findings.

'There are increasing numbers of young women and young men choosing more brutal ways to harm themselves. We are alarmed by the numbers being triggered into a drug-induced psychotic breakdown by the availability and society's tolerance of street drugs, particularly chemical hybrids like skunk, and alcohol. For those who are genetically or otherwise vulnerable, being pushed to flashpoint at an early age can lead to lifelong mental illness,' she said.

Griffiths said more resources, facilities and funding were desperately needed to combat the problems. 'As a society, we need to ask: do we value adolescence and can we create a culture in which young people can thrive? If not, can we live with the fallout?' he said.

Adolescent Angst from www. prioryhealthcare.co.uk.
29 November 2005

■ The above information is reprinted with kind permission from 0-19, published by Reed Business Information. For more information, please visit their website at www.0-19.co.uk.

Drug use, smoking and drinking

Drug use, smoking and drinking among young people in 2005 – headline figures

T he 2005 survey showed that around 11% of 11 to 15-year-olds had taken drugs in the last month, 9% had smoked at least one cigarette a week and 22% had drunk alcohol in the last week. The 2005 results were broadly similar to those in previous years.

Drug use

In 2005, 19% of pupils had taken drugs in the last year, a similar proportion to 2004 (18%) and a decrease from 21% in 2003.

As in previous years, prevalence of drug-taking increased with age: 6% of 11-year-olds had taken drugs in the last year compared with 34% of 15-year-olds.

In 2005, as in previous years, pupils were more likely to take cannabis than any other drug. Twelve per cent of pupils aged 11 to 15 had taken cannabis in the last year, a similar proportion to 2004 (11%). Prevalence in both 2005 and 2004 was lower than in 2003 (13%).

Smoking

The prevalence of regular smoking (at least one cigarette a week) in 2005 was 9%, the same as in 2004 and 2003 and a decrease from 10% in 2002. Girls are more likely to be regular smokers than boys (10% of girls compared with 7% of boys).

Drinking

The proportion of pupils who had never had a drink is the highest ever measured by this survey at 42% of pupils. However 22% had drunk alcohol in the last week.

■ Information from the Department of Health. Visit www.dh.gov.uk.

Young Brits lose stiff upper lip

But they still hide emotional secrets from friends

Young people look for comfort when they're upset or 'down' faster than any other age group, according to research carried out for Samaritans as part of its annual Winter Campaign. But they still have emotional 'secrets' they won't share with even their closest friends.

In a UK-wide survey of 2000 people the 15 to 24 year group come out on top when questioned if they'd been asked by a friend to talk over an emotional problem. 17 per cent of them said they would talk about a problem when it was only a day or two old; 38 per cent would talk it over within a week.

> *In a UK-wide survey of 2000 people the 15 to 24 year group come out on top when questioned if they'd been asked by a friend to talk over an emotional problem*

This contrasts greatly with the over 65s, many of whom prefer not to share emotional issues and say they do not look for support. 30 per cent of people who said they'd never reached out for emotional help were over 65.

A vital element of Samaritans' Winter Campaign – supported by the Vodafone UK Foundation – is showing young people, especially young men, who share problems less than women, that Samaritans is a 24/7 confidential and non-judgmental service for those problems you can't even talk to your closest friends about.

Consultant psychologist Dr Andrew McDowell of The Dream Mill Research said: 'Young people usually have a wide circle of friends, and then two or three who they are very close to but even they won't be let in on "secret problems". Things like family issues, abuse, domestic violence, or behaviour thought unacceptable within the group. These could vary from changing one drug used by friends to a "harder" drug or simply forming personal opinions you know would be unacceptable to your friends. This is where Samaritans plays such an important role – its volunteers provide a space to talk things through.'

More than half the people questioned found that the preferred ways of 'finding comfort' when upset were to spend time with family or talking to friends.

Find help 'on the big screen' – take time with a film

Samaritans' survey reveals 13% of men and women both hit the movies when they're feeling down … but better not forget the popcorn. 22 per cent of women find food a source of comfort; just three per cent choose sport.

More than one-third of people never seek help until problems are serious

Samaritans' research showed that 34% of people said they don't talk to anyone about an emotional problem until it becomes serious, or they never speak about it at all. Men are still less likely to talk over a problem straight away – 24 per cent of them doing so at once as against 34 per cent of women. As many as 25 per cent of men would wait until something is really serious before talking compared with 19 per cent of women.

A total of 16 per cent of men said they'd never talk over a problem they have – contrasting with nine per cent of women.

13 per cent of people questioned would call Samaritans for support.
29 November 2005

■ The above information is reprinted with kind permission from the Samaritans. Visit www.samaritans.org.uk for more information.

© Samaritans

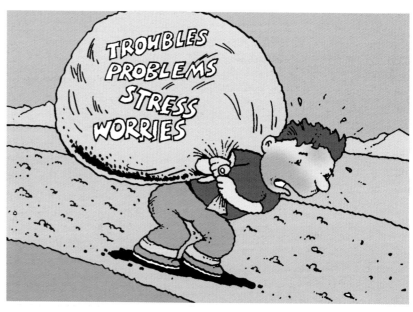

Young people and smoking

Information from Action on Smoking and Health (ASH)

Key facts

- About one in six boys and one in four girls are regular smokers by the age of 15.
- Children are three times more likely to smoke if their parents smoke.
- Two-thirds of teenage smokers say they would find it hard to go without cigarettes for a week.
- Half of smokers under the age of 16 who try to buy cigarettes from shops succeed in doing so.

About one in six boys and one in four girls are regular smokers by the age of 15

Smoking prevalence

Children become aware of cigarettes at an early age. Three out of four children are aware of cigarettes before they reach the age of five whether the parents smoke or not. The proportion of children who have experimented with smoking has fallen from 53% in 1982 to 39% in 2004. Since 1993, girls have been more likely than boys to have ever smoked. This contrasts with the results of regional studies of children's smoking habits during the 1960s and 1970s, which showed that more boys smoked than girls and that boys started earlier. In 1982, at ASH's instigation, the government commissioned the first national survey of smoking among children and found that 11% of 11 to 16-year-olds were smoking regularly.

During the early 1990s prevalence remained stable at 10%, but by the mid-1990s teenage smoking rates were on the increase, particularly among girls. Between 1996 and 1999, there was a decline in 11 to 15-year-olds smoking regularly. The reduction in smoking prevalence occurred mainly among 14 to 15-year-olds. In 1998, the government set a target to reduce the prevalence of regular smoking among young people aged 11 to 15 from a baseline of 13% in 1996 to 11% by 2005 and 9% or less by 2010. Results from the 2005 survey show no change in smoking prevalence since 2003. As in previous years, girls are more likely to be regular smokers than boys. The proportion of regular smokers increases sharply with age: 1% of 11-year-olds smoke regularly, compared with 20% of 15-year-olds.

What factors influence children to start smoking?

Children are three times as likely to smoke if both of their parents smoke and parents' approval or disapproval of the habit is also a significant factor. Numerous studies have shown that most young smokers are influenced by their friends' and older siblings' smoking habits. Surveys conducted before tobacco advertising was banned showed that children tended to smoke the brands that were promoted most heavily and that advertising reinforces the smoking habit. Advertising also creates the impression that smoking is a socially acceptable norm. Sports sponsorship by tobacco companies and particularly the televising of sponsored events increases children's awareness of the brands. A survey in 1996 found that around two-thirds of 11 to 16-year-olds could identify at least one sport connected to cigarette advertising through sponsorship. Another study found that boys whose favourite sport was motor racing were twice as likely to become regular smokers than those who did not have an interest in the sport.

Smoking and children's health

Children who smoke are two to six times more susceptible to coughs and increased phlegm, wheeziness and shortness of breath than those who do not smoke. Consequently, young smokers take more time off school than non-smokers. The earlier children become regular smokers and persist in the habit as adults, the greater the risk of developing lung cancer or heart disease. Smokers are also less fit than non-smokers: the performance in a half-marathon of a smoker of 20 cigarettes a day is that of a non-smoker 12 years older.

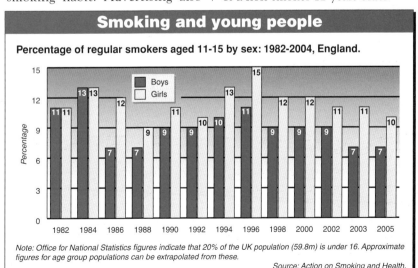

Smoking and young people

Percentage of regular smokers aged 11-15 by sex: 1982-2004, England.

Note: Office for National Statistics figures indicate that 20% of the UK population (59.8m) is under 16. Approximate figures for age group populations can be extrapolated from these.

Source: Action on Smoking and Health.

Children are also more susceptible to the effects of passive smoking. Parental smoking is the main determinant of exposure in non-smoking children. Although levels of exposure in the home have declined in the UK in recent years, children living in the poorest households have the highest levels of exposure as measured by cotinine, a marker for nicotine. (For further information about smoking in the home see ASH Factsheet no 25 'Secondhand Smoke in the Home'). Bronchitis, pneumonia, asthma and other chronic respiratory illnesses are significantly more common in infants and children who have one or two smoking parents. Children of parents who smoke during the child's early life run a higher risk of cancer in adulthood and the larger the number of smokers in a household, the greater the cancer risk to non-smokers in the family. For a more detailed overview of the health impacts of passive smoking on children see the ASH briefing: 'Passive smoking: the impact on children.'

Addiction

Children who experiment with cigarettes quickly become addicted to the nicotine in tobacco. A MORI survey of children aged 11 to 16 years found that teenagers have similar levels of nicotine dependence as adults, with one-third of those who smoke one or more cigarettes a week lighting up their first cigarette within 30 minutes of waking up and one in 12 lighting up within the first five minutes. In 2004, 66% of smokers aged 11 to 15 reported that they would find it difficult to go without smoking for a week, while 79% thought they would find it difficult to give up altogether. During periods of abstinence, young people experience withdrawal symptoms similar to the kind experienced by adult smokers.

One-third of teenagers who smoke one or more cigarettes a week light up their first cigarette within 30 minutes of waking up and one in 12 light up within the first five minutes

---

Smoking prevention

Since the 1970s, health education including information about the health effects of smoking has been included in the curricula of most primary and secondary schools in Great Britain. Research suggests that knowledge about smoking is a necessary component of anti-smoking campaigns but by itself does not affect smoking rates. It may, however, result in a postponement of initiation. High prices can deter children from smoking, since they do not possess a large disposable income. In Canada, when cigarette prices were raised dramatically in the 1980s and the early 1990s, youth consumption of tobacco plummeted by 60%. An American study has shown that while price does not appear to affect initial experimentation of smoking, it is an important tool in reducing youth smoking once the habit has become established.

Children, smoking and the law

Since 1908, and currently under the Children and Young Persons (Protection from Tobacco) Act 1991, it has been illegal to sell any tobacco product to anyone below the age of 16. The Act increased the maximum fines for retailers found guilty of selling cigarettes to children to £2,500 and prohibited the sale of single cigarettes. Despite the law, children still succeed in buying tobacco from shops and vending machines. During 2003 there were 117 prosecutions in England and Wales for underage tobacco sales, with 93 defendants being found guilty and 82 fined. Of these, 26 fines were for sums over £300.

Between 1986 and 1996, the proportion of children aged 11 to 15 trying to buy cigarettes from a shop fluctuated between 24% and 32%. Since then it has been gradually decreasing and was 17% in 2004. Of these, 52% of teenagers had been refused on at least one occasion. Legislation alone is not sufficient to prevent tobacco sales to minors. Both enforcement and community policies may improve compliance by retailers, but the impact on underage smoking prevalence using these approaches alone may still be small. Successful efforts to limit underage access to tobacco require a combination of approaches that tackle the problem comprehensively.
April 2006

■ The above information is reprinted with kind permission from Action on Smoking and Health. For more information and references, please visit the Action on Smoking and Health website at www.ash.org.uk.
© *Action on Smoking and Health*

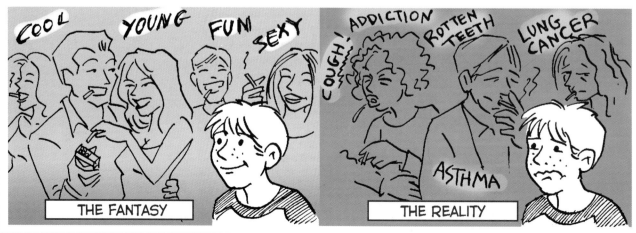

THE FANTASY — COOL YOUNG FUN SEXY

THE REALITY — COUGH! ADDICTION ROTTEN TEETH LUNG CANCER ASTHMA

Smoking and the 'sleeper effect'

'Sleeper effect' leaves children vulnerable to starting smoking years after single cigarette

Children's vulnerability to taking up smoking after trying just a single cigarette can lie dormant for three years or more – according to a new study from Cancer Research UK published today in the journal *Tobacco Control*.

The researchers conclude that this lasting predisposition – or 'sleeper effect' – may mean it is important to prevent young adolescents from trying even one cigarette.

Children who smoked just one cigarette by the age of 11 were more than twice as likely to take up smoking over the next few years as those who did not experiment with smoking

---

Also, that young people who have tried smoking just once a number of years previously, should be considered as a key target group for prevention messages and anti-smoking support.

The study of teenage smoking behaviour found that children who smoked just one cigarette by the age of 11 were more than twice as likely to take up smoking over the next few years as those who did not experiment with smoking – even after a gap of up to three years of not smoking.

The findings held true even once factors known to influence the chances of taking up smoking – such as gender, ethnicity, deprivation and parental smoking – were taken into consideration.

The team tracked the smoking behaviour of over 2,000 London schoolchildren aged 11 to 16 over five years and measured their nicotine intake by analysing their saliva.

Of the 260 children who, at age 11, said they had tried smoking just once, 18 per cent were smokers at age 14. In comparison, seven per cent of children who, at age 11, said they had never smoked had started smoking by age 14.

Lead researcher Jennifer Fidler, who is based at the Cancer Research UK Health Behaviour Unit at University College London, said:

'We know that progression from experimenting with one cigarette to being a smoker can take several years. But for the first time we've shown that there may be a period of dormancy between trying cigarettes and becoming a regular smoker – a "sleeper effect" or vulnerability to nicotine addiction.

This has important practical and policy implications. It may be that preventing children from trying even one cigarette is a much more important goal than first thought. And that prevention efforts might be most effective if focused on pre-secondary school children.'

Jennifer Fidler added: 'The results also indicate that prior experimentation is a strong predictor of taking up smoking later. And the finding of a "sleeper effect" suggests that health care providers designing targeted campaigns should focus on young teenagers who report having tried cigarettes in the past.'

There are several possible explanations for this 'sleeper effect', say the authors. Pathways in the brain may become changed as a consequence of a single exposure to nicotine, increasing vulnerability to smoking triggers such as stress,

depression or the school environment at a later date. Or experimenting with a cigarette might break down barriers that would otherwise prevent teenagers from taking up smoking – such as insecurities about how to smoke and fear of being caught by adults.

Jean King, director of tobacco control at Cancer Research UK, said: 'This study is particularly important because, in 2004, 14 per cent of 11-year-olds and 62 per cent of 15-year-olds in England said they had experimented with cigarettes.

'Smoking is the single biggest preventable cause of cancer in the UK. And we know that there's a "hard-to-reach" group of young smokers that anti-smoking campaigns are failing to connect with. Any research that helps unravel the processes involved in young people becoming addicted to nicotine is key to developing effective and targeted ways to prevent them from starting smoking in the first place.'

24 May 2006

■ The above information is reprinted with kind permission from Cancer Research UK. Visit www.cancerresearchuk.org for more information.

Drugs and alcohol

Mental health and growing up

Introduction

Lots of young people want to know about drugs and alcohol. However much willpower you have, it is very easy to end up finding you have a problem. Although you may initially think that you have your drug or alcohol use 'under control', these things can be very addictive and may soon start to control you.

Commonly used drugs

People use all sorts of substances, both legal and illegal. The obviously illegal drugs are things like cannabis (hash), speed (amphetamines), ecstasy (E), cocaine and heroin. Many legal substances are also harmful and addictive – cigarettes, alcohol, glue, petrol and aerosols. Society's favourite drugs are alcohol and tobacco, both strongly addictive and misused by millions. A few medicines, such as tranquillisers, can also be addictive.

Although you may initially think that you have your drug or alcohol use 'under control', these things can be very addictive and may soon start to control you

What leads to problems with drugs and alcohol?

- You may worry that if you don't take drugs, you will be 'uncool' and won't fit in.
- Drugs can make you feel good for a while. Just experimenting with a drug may make you want to try again ... and again.
- You find that taking a particular drug makes you feel confident, and may help you to face a difficult situation. After a while, you need the drug to face that situation every time.

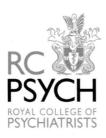

RC PSYCH
ROYAL COLLEGE OF PSYCHIATRISTS

- If you are unhappy, stressed, or lonely, you are more likely to turn to drugs to forget your problems.
- If you find that you're using a drug or alcohol more and more often, be careful – this is the first step to becoming dependent on it.
- If you hang out with people who use a lot of drugs, you probably will too.

Risks and dangers

Using street drugs or alcohol might make you feel good, but they can damage your health. Here are some of the basic facts.

- It is dangerous to mix drugs and alcohol. They each may increase the effects of the other substance, e.g. ecstasy and alcohol can lead to dehydration (overheating), and cause coma and death.
- You cannot know for sure what is in the drug you buy. It might not contain what the dealer says. Some dealers might mix it with other substances or you may get a higher dose of a drug than you are used to, which can be fatal.
- Serious infections can be spread by sharing needles or 'equipment', such as HIV and hepatitis.
- Accidents, arguments and fights are more likely after drinking and drug use.
- Using drugs can lead to serious mental illness such as psychosis or depression, and to health problems and overdoses.

Signs that you're hooked

- Do you think about drugs or alcohol everyday?
- Is it hard to say 'no' when they are offered?

- Would you drink/take drugs alone?
- Does taking drugs get in the way of the rest of your life?

If the answer to these questions is 'yes', you may be hooked.

The most common sign that you have a drug problem is the feeling the drug gives you suddenly, it's not a choice that feels under your control. Soon, you'll find yourself having to take drugs more and more to get the same effect. Then, you'll find that you can't cope without it and that you've got a habit, although you'll find yourself saying: 'It's not that I need it, but ...'

How to get help

There are different ways of getting help. Think about talking to someone you trust, such as:

- a close friend;
- your parents or a family member;
- a family friend;
- a school nurse;
- a social worker;
- a teacher/school counsellor;
- someone at your place of worship;
- a youth counsellor;
- your GP or practice nurse, who can refer you on to relevant services, and will be able to offer you advice and support;
- a local drug project. See your local area telephone book or ask for the address from your health centre;
- your local child and adolescent mental health service – this is a team of skilled professionals, including child psychiatrists, psychologists, social workers, psychotherapists and specialist nurses.

- The above information is reprinted with kind permission from the Royal College of Psychiatrists. For more information, please visit their website at www.rcpsych.ac.uk.

Alcohol facts for young people

Information from Surgery Door

Introduction

So what does being drunk mean to you?

- trolleyed;
- sozzled;
- leathered;
- lagged;
- paralytic;
- plastered;
- legless;
- tanked-up;
- bladdered;
- bevvied;
- pissed;
- hammered;
- squiffy;
- tipsy;
- Brahms and Liszt;
- slaughtered;
- blotto;
- pie-eyed;
- slashed;
- off yer face;
- wrecked;
- blasted.

'They just show off and try to act macho. It's pathetic.' Kate, 14
'It's when other people in your group think, "What an idiot!"' Paul, 18
'It gets annoying sometimes when the girls just sit there giggling together at everything you say.' Pete, 17
'She was crying her eyes out and said, "you hate me". It's stupid – she's my best friend!' Sally, 14
'If alcohol disappeared, there'd be no way to enjoy yourself.' Mike, 17

The good, the bad, the ugly

We all like a laugh. And you can't have a laugh on a night out if you're not going to have a drink or several, can you?

Trouble is, with alcohol there's no off-switch if you decide you've had too much.

You're with a group and you're drinking rounds, or maybe sharing a bottle or a six pack. You're drinking quickly – keeping up with your mates.

Before you know it, you're feeling really rough. So you have another drink, hoping you'll feel better. And pretty soon you're not feeling much at all.

Except when you wake up the next day and can't remember how you got there or what you did. And how scary is that?

There are loads of reasons for not getting completely trashed. For starters:

- you're more likely to make a hit with someone you're keen to impress if you're being yourself;
- you'll be able to look out for your mates if things get out of hand;
- you might avoid doing something you'll regret. Like getting off with Mr or Miss Personality Bypass, or having sex when you don't really want to, or not bothering to use a condom;
- no more throwing your guts up all night;
- you'll get home safely and getting up won't be so bad;
- you'll feel and look better. Unless your idea of attractive is a blotchy face, bloodshot eyes, a furry tongue, and depressed to boot;
- you'll be fitter. Drinking damages the muscle fibres you need for sports;
- you won't blow all your cash on an evening out you can't remember.

The other side of the bottle

Alcohol can affect you in all kinds of ways – even if you're not the one drinking it.

'My dad is alcohol dependent, he carries a litre of whisky. The fact that my dad drinks is scary and makes me think he's pathetic.' Sue, 18

More than two million people in Britain grow up in families where one or both parents have a drink problem. You may be one of them or you may know someone in that situation. You're not on your own – we can tell you where to go for confidential advice and information.

It's time to take action!

The next section looks at everything you need to know about alcohol – whether you have already tried it, you think you'll try it in the future or you never plan to drink.

Get it right!

If you're planning on drinking, it's important to know how alcohol is going to affect you. That way you can stay in control of your drink – rather than the other way around.

Alcohol gets into the bloodstream within a few minutes of drinking and is carried to all parts of the body. The effects can take hours to wear off and vary depending on:

- how much and how quickly a person is drinking;
- what they've been drinking (stronger drinks like spirits and fizzy drinks like cider are absorbed more quickly);
- how used they are to drinking alcohol;
- their size and weight.

If a person is smaller or lighter, the alcohol will be concentrated into a smaller body volume. So alcohol will affect a person who isn't fully grown more quickly.

It's a biological fact – drink for drink, alcohol will affect a woman more than a man. Women are generally smaller, their bodies contain less water and their metabolism is different.

Alcohol affects physical coordination, reaction times and decision-making.

People who are drunk are more likely to have an accident, get into arguments or take stupid risks. They may feel sick, have blackouts or lose consciousness.

Drinking alcohol together with taking illegal drugs is particularly dangerous, increasing the likelihood of a serious drug overdose.

How much are you really drinking?

All alcoholic drinks contain pure alcohol (ethanol) in varying amounts.

Their strength is shown on the label by a number followed by Alcohol %vol, %vol or %ABV. The higher the percentage, the stronger the drink.

Alcohol can also be measured in units. One unit is equivalent to 10ml (1cl) of pure alcohol.

Each of the following contains one unit:
- a half pint of ordinary strength lager/beer/cider (3.5% ABV);
- a small glass of wine (9% ABV) Note: many wines are 11 or 12% ABV;
- a 25ml pub measure of spirit.

If a young person is going to drink, they should drink well below the benchmarks for fully-grown adults. These adult benchmarks are: between three and four units or fewer in any day when alcohol is drunk for men and between two and three units or fewer for women.

The hard facts

When you're thinking of drinking, keep the following in mind.
- Around half of all pedestrians aged 16 to 60 killed in road accidents have more booze in their bloodstream than the legal drink-drive limit.
- 1,000 children under the age of 15 are admitted to hospital each year with acute alcohol poisoning.
- All need emergency treatment.
- Around half of all adults admitted to hospital with head injuries are drunk.
- Alcohol is a factor in at least 7% of accidental drownings and 40% of household fires.
- You can get a criminal record for offences of drunkenness. Being drunk will be no excuse if you

end up in court on a charge of criminal damage or violence.
- In 1994, 57,800 people were found guilty or cautioned for drunkenness. The peak age of offenders was 18.

Some types of drink preferred by young people are much stronger than average, for example strong beers and ciders. There can be as much alcohol in a 330ml bottle of alcopop as in a generous shot of whisky.

What to do in an emergency

It is important to know what to do if someone becomes unconscious after drinking too much alcohol.
- Dial 999 straight away and ask for an ambulance.
- Never feel too ashamed to involve the emergency services.
- Place them in the recovery position so they won't choke if they vomit.
- Check their breathing. Be prepared to do mouth-to-mouth resuscitation.
- Keep them warm, but not too hot.
- Stay with them at all times. If you need to leave to call an ambulance, go straight back.

If someone becomes unconscious they should be gently moved into the recovery position so their tongue cannot fall back and prevent breathing.

If someone is heavily under the influence of alcohol, don't leave them to sleep it off alone. There is a risk of choking if they vomit. Keep an eye on them, make sure they sleep on their side, and check that they keep breathing.

What the law says

Under five
It is illegal to give an alcoholic drink to a child under five except under medical supervision in an emergency.

Under 14
You cannot go into the bar of a pub unless it has a 'children's certificate'. If it does not have one, you can only go into parts of licensed premises where alcohol is either sold but not drunk (e.g. a sales point for consumption away from the pub), or drunk but not sold (e.g. a garden or family room).

14 or 15
You can go anywhere in a pub, but not drink alcohol.

16 or 17
You can buy or be bought beer or cider to drink with a meal, but not in a bar (i.e. in an area specifically set aside for meals).

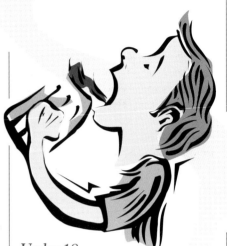

Under 18
Except for 16- or 17-year-olds having a meal in a pub (see above), it is against the law for anyone under 18 to buy alcohol in a pub, off-licence, supermarket or other outlet, or for anyone to buy alcohol in a pub for someone under 18.

Some towns and cities have local bye-laws banning drinking alcohol in public.

Tips for talking

Conversations about alcohol can all too easily turn into lectures, accusations or rows. But remember, young people and parents can both gain from having calm discussions.

Discussions will be easier if:
- parents show that their main concern is their child's health, safety and well-being;
- you both try to explain your feelings and listen carefully to each other's point of view;
- you talk with each other, not at each other;
- you are both prepared to come to a compromise.

At what age should a young person start drinking?

Parents may be concerned about:
- their child's safety;
- the possible effects of alcohol;

- their child being pressurised by friends;
- strong beliefs about not drinking alcohol.

A young person may:
- be curious about alcohol;
- not want to be left out;
- want to drink alcohol because their friends say that their parents let them;
- want to do something that adults do.

The common ground here could be: the young person reaching 21 without being rushed to hospital, and without being left out by their friends.

Parties at home?

Before having a party, it's important for young people and parents to set some ground rules.

Possible issues to talk about and agree on include the following.
- Is alcohol going to be provided? If so, what types?

Around half of all adults admitted to hospital with head injuries are drunk

- How will the young person/parent deal with partygoers who bring drinks that you've agreed won't be available?
- What can be done to help prevent drink-related trouble?
- Will the party be open house or by invite only?
- Should parents be around – but in the background?
- Who will clear up and when?

By agreeing ground rules, the young person and their friends can have a good time, without their parents having a nervous breakdown.

Getting home safely after a night out

A young person and their parents could make a pact which is agreeable to both parties.

Your pact could be:
- neither will drive if they have been drinking;
- neither will be a passenger if the driver has been drinking;
- the young person will not spend their cab fare home on other things;

- the young person will tell their parent where they are going;
- the parent will try not to interfere in the young person's social life.

Getting further information and advice

Alcohol Concern
020 7928 7377 – For general information about alcohol.

National Alcohol Helpline
0800 917 8282 – All calls are free. For confidential information, help and advice if you are worried about a young person's drinking, the drinking of someone else in the family, or your own drinking.

Al-Anon Family Groups
020 7403 0888 – For the families of people with drinking problems.

Alateen Groups
020 7403 0888 – For teenagers in families where someone has a drinking problem.

Contact your local health promotion unit or alcohol advisory service for general information about alcohol. You'll find their number in the phone book.

The Health Education Authority produces a range of leaflets about alcohol, including:
- 'A Parent's Guide to Drugs and Alcohol';
- 'Say when... how much is too much?';
- 'Think about drink';
- 'Your Drink and You' – a leaflet targeting the Caribbean community;
- 'Alcohol: The Facts' – a leaflet aimed at South-Asian adults .

To order copies of any of these leaflets phone Marston Book Services on 01235 465500. Your local health promotion unit (in the phone book under Health Promotion Unit or Health Education Unit) may also have copies.

- Information from Surgery Door. Visit www.surgerydoor.co.uk for more information.

© Surgery Door

Substance misuse

The facts

- The Department of Health estimates that 47% of 15-year-olds have drunk alcohol in the last week, and 22% have used an illegal drug.
- At least one million children in the UK are living in a family home where problematic alcohol use is an issue.
- 27% of 11 to 15-year-olds have used an illicit drug in the last month.
- Approximately 300,000 children live in a home where heroin or crack is used (3% of all children).
- 35% of all child protection enquiries feature heroin or crack.
- Up to 50% of all crime is drug-related.
- Secondary school-age children, particularly older children, are commonly offered illegal drugs. Children who do not themselves use drugs or alcohol are quite likely to know someone who does.
- Over 500,000 ecstasy tablets are taken every weekend, an increasing amount by children and young people.
- One in 12 of 12-year-olds have tried drugs at least once, this increases to one in three of 14-year-olds and two in five of 16-year-olds.
- Re-Solv, a campaign and education group funded by the solvents industry, estimates that one-third of all volatile substance-related deaths occur the first time the substance is used – casualties are virtually all children.
- Some police forces estimate that up to 70% of all crime is drug or alcohol-related. It is estimated that alcohol is a feature in 80% of incidences of domestic violence, and 40% of child abuse.

- The above information is reprinted with kind permission from Barnardo's. Visit www.barnardos.org.uk for more information.

© Barnardo's

Wide eyed and legless

Information from *0-19*, published by Reed Business Information

At the end of August, Mark Shields from Northumberland was found dead in bed on the morning of his 18th birthday after celebrating the night before with five pints of lager, five double whiskies and three double shots of liqueur in less than 40 minutes. This tragedy followed the revelation that, in 2003-2004, 13 teenagers a day were admitted to hospital suffering from the affects of alcohol abuse.

It is unsurprising then that alcohol charities, doctors, the Association of Chief Police Officers and judges have all expressed serious concerns about next month's introduction of relaxed licensing laws, which will allow pubs and bars to open around the clock.

The list of problems alcohol causes young people is long and ranges from health-related issues, to behaviour and relationship problems, to a heightened risk of being the victim or the perpetrator of violence.

'When we see young people in Accident and Emergency as a result of violence, in the vast majority of cases alcohol is involved,' says Dr Vivienne Nathanson, head of science and ethics at the British Medical Association, who warns that we are facing a public health epidemic. 'We are going to see an explosion of serious liver disease in young adults and that's very worrying. The consequences for individuals and society will be catastrophic.'

Her concerns are echoed by Dr Clare Gerada, a south-London GP and director of the Substance Misuse Unit at the Royal College of General Practitioners.

'Disinhibition caused by drink is a major issue for young people and places them at greater risk of making bad decisions like having unprotected sex or taking drugs,' she says. 'It isn't necessarily now that we are going to see the health problems of 14 to 15-year-old drinkers – our worry as doctors is that we are sitting on a potential explosion of alcohol-related problems in 10 years' time.

'We don't know what alcohol – and particularly spirits – is going to do to their young livers and their young brains.'

Alcohol charity Alcohol Concern says there is a lot of work to be done in turning around attitudes to alcohol, and in talking to young people about the issues. 'The worrying trend for us is that young people are drinking much greater quantities and more frequently,' says Geethika Jayatilaka, director of policy and public affairs at the charity.

'There are links between alcohol and early sex – which is sometimes regretted – and we have found that alcohol played a part in 20% of school exclusions.'

Jayatilaka stresses that it's really important to get the tone and message of education and information

right and to make sure the messages resonate for young people, who are likely to be facing peer pressure.

'We know that there is a certain amount of ambivalence in communicating the messages around alcohol because 90% of people drink themselves. We need to give teachers and youth workers the skills and confidence to talk about the issues without feeling awkward or hypocritical,' she says.

Nathanson wants to see the government look closely at all the factors that encourage young people to drink. 'We need a joined-up approach to the problem with education as a key plank and that needs to start in schools,' she says.

A quarter of pupils who had drunk in the last week had consumed 14 units or more

---

Gerada, meanwhile, cautions against demonising young people, saying that they simply echo what adults do. 'We should stop making it their problem – it's not theirs, it's ours,' she says.

The Scottish Executive seems to have taken this message to heart. In March this year it published the Licensing (Scotland) Bill to tackle the country's 'shocking' record on alcohol. The measures will call time on happy hour and other 'irresponsible' drink promotions, and sales drives designed to appeal to young people will be banned in supermarkets and off-licences.

As 24/7 drinking becomes a reality in Britain next month, many will be hoping that Westminster will consider following Scotland's lead.

Factfile
1. Alcohol-related deaths have risen by nearly one fifth in the last four years.

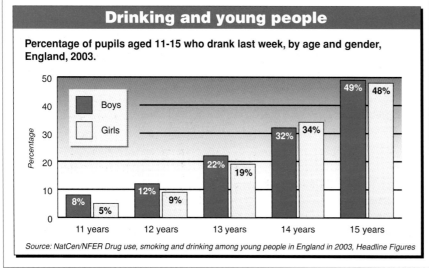

Drinking and young people

Percentage of pupils aged 11-15 who drank last week, by age and gender, England, 2003.

- Boys
- Girls

	11 years	12 years	13 years	14 years	15 years
Boys	8%	12%	22%	32%	49%
Girls	5%	9%	19%	34%	48%

Source: NatCen/NFER Drug use, smoking and drinking among young people in England in 2003, Headline Figures

2. The real price of alcohol has halved in the UK since the 1960s.

3. A major NHS survey of 11 to 15-year-old schoolchildren published in August found that:
   - nearly half of 15-year-old pupils had drunk alcohol in the last week;
   - a quarter of pupils who had drunk in the last week had consumed 14 units or more;
   - more young people are drinking spirits and alcopops – although beer, lager and cider were still the most popular overall;
   - nearly half those surveyed had been drunk in the last week;
   - nearly one third deliberately tried to get drunk.

'There's no one stereotype'

Branching Out is a joint venture between Lifeline and Turning Point and offers a multi-agency service to young people aged under 19 who are using, or at risk of using, drugs and alcohol in the Tameside and Glossop areas of the north.

Team leader Emma Hawley says: 'We get referrals from the Youth Offending Team, the Connexions service, social services and, more and more often, people self-refer.'

She stresses that the young people come from all sorts of backgrounds. 'Some are involved in offending, but not all; some are in education, some are not; some are very much engaged with their families and for others there is a difficult family relationship. There's no one stereotype.'

The catalyst for a referral varies, but Hawley says that quite often it is when the young person realises that they have a problem. 'Parents might be laying down the law, or it might be that they are involved with the Youth Offending Team and that alcohol was a factor in them committing their offence. Some of the young people have mental health problems and seek help when they reach some sort of crisis.

'We work with them to help them resolve their problems with alcohol and this will be different with every young person ranging from stopping using altogether through to reducing their use or using more safely.'

Hawley adds that parents often need support too to deal with the conflict that can arise as a result of the stress of having a child who drinks too much. 'They might be having problems with curfews; the impact the drinking is having on schoolwork; and general behaviour problems,' says Hawley. 'Quite often parents just need someone to talk to and get advice from outside of their own families.'

1 October 2005

- Information from *0-19*, published by Reed Business Information. For more information, please visit their website at www.0-19.co.uk.

© Reed Business Information

What teens really think about sex

Experts shocked as report reveals depths of ignorance that lead many to unsafe sex

Eight out of 10 teenagers lose their virginity when they are drunk, feeling pressurised into having sex or are not using contraception, a survey has revealed.

The research, conducted by the Trust for the Study of Adolescence, will alarm government ministers, who are concerned that the UK has the highest rate of teenage pregnancy in western Europe and that sexually-transmitted infections (STIs), such as chlamydia, are found mainly in those aged 16 to 19.

The survey of 3,000 London secondary school pupils aged 15 to 18 found that:
- 39 per cent had sex for the first time when one or other partner was not equally willing;
- almost three in 10 lost their virginity for 'negative reasons',

By Denis Campbell,
Social Affairs Correspondent

such as wanting to please a boyfriend;
- 51 per cent of girls and 37 per cent of boys had had unprotected sex;
- 58 per cent of girls and 39 per cent of boys had slept with someone at least once without using a condom;
- two in five wish they had waited longer before having sex;
- only 20 per cent who have sex for the first time take precautions, are in a steady relationship or feel the timing is right.

Anna Martinez of the Sex Education Forum said. 'These results show that there's a lot of ignorance among young people about sex and that too many are becoming involved in high-risk sexual behaviour before they have had the chance to learn about issues such as how to resist pressure from partners, friends and the media to have sex. Schools, parents and professionals are failing young people by not giving them adequate support and information.'

The Trust's report, carried out for the Naz sexual health project in west London, reveals for the first time how sexual attitudes and experiences vary between ethnic groups. While 80 per cent of all the teenagers surveyed were 'not sexually competent' the first time they had sex, that figure rose to 93 per cent for boys of black Caribbean origin, for example. And 32 per cent of boys of black African origin did not use contraception when they first had sex, compared to 10 per cent of white British pupils and 18 per cent of interviewees overall.

Many of those from ethnic minority backgrounds knew little about how to prevent and identify the symptoms of STIs, and black Caribbean young men were more likely than others to have risky sex.

Bryan Teixeira, chief executive of the Naz project, said many young people from ethnic minority backgrounds ended up confused about sex because, while their parents often have traditional views, sex was discussed openly at school. Boys and young men were a particular problem, said Teixeira, as they were more likely to indulge in risky sexual behaviour and to have more partners than girls.

Just 18 per cent of respondents had had sex before 16, the age of consent, which contradicts the impression of widespread underage sex

---

Although few places have as many pupils from an ethnic minority background as the Londoners in the survey – well over half – the results paint a worrying picture of the sex lives of Britain's 5.2 million teenagers.

However, just 18 per cent of respondents had had sex before 16, the age of consent, which contradicts the impression of widespread underage sex and shows no increase on statistics from previous studies.

The report's call for sex and relationships education to be made compulsory in schools to help tackle what Teixeira calls 'widespread knowledge gaps' and to help pupils ensure their sexual welfare, was backed by *CosmoGIRL* magazine, which has been running a high-profile 'Just Say Know' campaign.

Editor Celia Duncan said: 'Some of the findings in this report are shocking and underline the case for all secondary school pupils to be taught not just about how to create a baby, but also about how to handle a guy who is pressurising you to have sex.

'There are too many myths bandied about in the playground, such as 'you can't get pregnant your first time'. If pupils remain ignorant about sex, the consequences will be higher rates of STIs and unwanted pregnancies.'

A £50m Department of Health advertising campaign promoting responsible sex is due to start this autumn.

A teenager's view

Bethany Cole, a 16-year-old schoolgirl from Buckingham, thinks there is still not enough sex education.

'Most people I know haven't had sex yet and didn't have sex before turning 16. They don't care about breaking the law as they think no one will find out. Some male friends joke about sex and say that they've "had it", but I suspect much of that is just male bravado. Me and my girlfriends do talk about sex; for example, if someone has had sex for the first time with a new boyfriend, or asks us if she can catch a sexually-transmitted infection from something she did at the weekend. But my friends are pretty responsible, and use condoms, for example.

'I'm lucky. I got a lot of sex education at school. Our form tutor gave one lesson over to answering questions that we'd all submitted anonymously, to minimise the embarrassment, which taught me a lot. Like how you can catch an STI or know if you've got one, and how to deal with peers or boyfriends who are pressuring you to have sex.

'It's crazy that many other schools, including one near mine, don't give education on sex and relationships. It should be compulsory at all secondary schools – there'd be fewer teenage pregnancies, STIs and infertility caused by people leaving an STI untreated.

'Some people say that if you teach young people about sex they'll be more likely to do it. But I've been taught about the dangers of smoking since I was 12 and haven't been tempted to try that. Proper sex education clues you up.'
21 May 2006

■ This article first appeared in *The Observer*.

© Guardian Newspapers Limited 2006

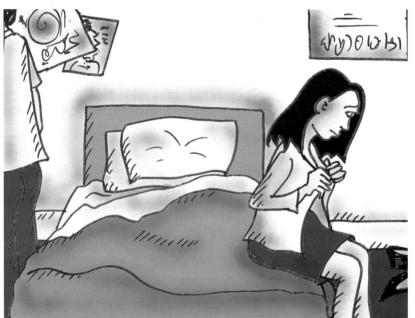

Teenage sexual activity

Information from Brook

First sexual experience

The age at which young people today report their first experience of sex is 14 for women and 13 for men.

First sexual intercourse

The age at which the majority of 16 to 19-year-olds today first have sexual intercourse is 16. Almost 30% of young men and almost 26% of young women report having intercourse before their 16th birthday. By the age of 20 the vast majority of young people today have had sexual intercourse.

Homosexual experience

Among 16 to 24-year-olds, 4% of men and 9% of women report some homosexual experience, with 5% and 10% respectively saying they have experienced homosexual attraction.

Trends in sexual behaviour

There has been a sharp drop in the age at first intercourse over the last 50 years. 26% of young women today experience sexual intercourse before the age of 16 compared with fewer than 1% of those who were young in the 1950s. Among young men, 30% report intercourse before 16 compared with 6% of men in the 1950s.

The age at first sexual experience has also dropped years from 16 to 14 for women and from 15 to 13 for men. However the time between first experience and first intercourse is shortening, particularly for women. Young women today now have intercourse about two years after their first sexual experience compared with four years during the 1950s.

Is the pill responsible for young people having sex earlier?

The biggest drop in age at first intercourse, from 21 to 19, occurred during the 1950s. The age of first intercourse fell as much during this one decade as it did over the next 30 years. This was before the introduction of the pill in 1961, which did not become widely available to unmarried women until 1972.

Reasons for first intercourse

Young people cite natural follow-on, being in love and curiosity as the main reasons why they had first intercourse. Although young men are more likely to say they had intercourse out of curiosity and women because they are in love, there has been a steady convergence between the sexes on the reasons for first intercourse.

Peer pressure

Although the majority of young people do not report having first intercourse because of peer pressure, young men are more likely than women to cite pressure from peers as the main reason for losing their virginity. Among teenage women claiming they were pressurised into first intercourse, 82% said the pressure came from boyfriends.

Feelings about first intercourse

Among 16 to 24-year-olds, 20% of men and 42% of women felt they had intercourse too soon. The younger the age at first intercourse, the more likely the regret.

Factors associated with first intercourse under 16

Educational achievements: median age at first intercourse increases with educational level. Young people reaching at least GCSE standard education are less likely to have intercourse before the age of 16.

Sex education: young people who cite friends and the media as their main sources of information about sex have first sexual intercourse younger than those who report school sex education as their main source.

Socio-economic status: young people whose parents are manual workers are more likely to have early intercourse than the children of non-manual workers as are young people who do not live with both parents.

Early sexual experience: the earlier the age of first sexual experience, the younger the age at first intercourse.

Early menarche: women who first menstruate at 13 or older are much less likely to have sex under 16 than those who start their periods under 13.

Patterns of sexual relationships

The vast majority of young people have their first sexual intercourse in an established relationship.

Young people are increasingly likely to plan their first sexual intercourse. As planned intercourse is more likely to be protected, this trend is likely to increase contraceptive use among teenagers.

Fewer than 1% of young people are married at the time of first sexual intercourse. Serial monogamy is still the most common pattern of sexual relationships among young people.

The percentage of young men having their first sexual intercourse with a prostitute has steadily declined over the last 40 years. This was reported by 3.4% of men who were young in the 1950s compared with 0% of young men today.

International comparisons

The age at which young people today report having first sexual intercourse does not vary significantly between developed countries.

■ The above information is an extract from a Brook factsheet and is reprinted with permission. Brook provides free and confidential sexual health advice and services specifically for young people under 25. For references and further information, visit www.brook.org.uk or contact the Young People's Information Service by calling 0800 0185 023 or texting BROOK HELP to 81222.

© *Brook Advisory Centres*

Birth control and contraception for teenagers

Information from AVERT

What is birth control?

Birth control means things you can do to ensure that pregnancy only happens if and when you want it to.

Birth control can mean abstinence. Abstinence is deciding not to do something, and abstaining from having sexual intercourse will ensure that pregnancy does not occur.

Birth control can also mean using a method of contraception to ensure that pregnancy does not occur when you do have sexual intercourse.

What causes a girl to become pregnant?

If a girl gets semen (the fluid released by a man's penis when he ejaculates or 'comes') inside or even just around her vagina, this can make her pregnant. This is because semen contains sperm. Pre-cum (the white liquid that leaks out of a man's erect penis before he ejaculates) can also contain sperm and therefore can also cause pregnancy. The most usual way semen and pre-cum get in or around the vagina is during sexual intercourse: when a boy's hard penis goes inside a girl's vagina. (There is more information on the AVERT website about having sexual intercourse for the first time).

Usually, sometime between the ages of 11 and 15, a girl begins to have periods. This shows that the ovaries have begun to produce eggs. An egg is released every month. If it does not meet up with the sperm that comes out of the boy's penis during intercourse, it dies. Then it leaves the body in the blood which comes out through the vagina during a girl's period every month.

If a girl has sexual intercourse with a boy and neither of them uses contraception, then the girl could become pregnant and a baby will begin to grow inside her womb.

AVERT

AVERTing HIV & AIDS Worldwide

A girl can become pregnant:
- even if she has sex standing up;
- the first time she has sex;
- even if she has sex during her period;
- even if a boy pulls out (or withdraws) before he comes;
- if she forgets to take her pill.

If you have sexual intercourse, pregnancy can be prevented by using a reliable method of contraception.

Birth control can mean abstinence. Abstinence is deciding not to do something, and abstaining from having sexual intercourse will ensure that pregnancy does not occur

---

Are there many different methods of contraception?

How do you know which one to choose?

Where do you get contraceptives from?

There are a number of different methods of contraception, all of which have their individual advantages and disadvantages. So as there is no clearly best method you have to decide which is most suitable for you. All forms of contraception work by preventing the fertilisation

of a woman's egg by a man's sperm. This can be achieved in various ways.

The first type are the barrier methods, which physically prevent sperm from swimming into the uterus and fertilising the woman's egg. The second type are hormonal methods which alter a woman's hormonal cycle to prevent fertilisation. These are the only types of contraception which are generally used by teenagers.

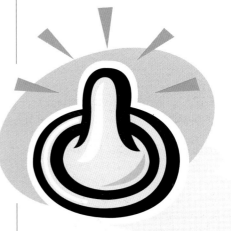

Other types of contraception which are generally not used by young people include the intrauterine device (IUD), which is generally not recommended for young women who have not had children; natural methods, which are often not effective enough; and sterilisation which is a permanent surgical procedure.

All the hormonal methods of contraception are only available from a doctor. Some barrier methods such as the IUD are also only available from a doctor, but others such as the male condom and spermicides are widely available in most countries. Another great advantage of barrier methods of contraception is that, if used properly every time, they also provide effective protection against sexually-transmitted diseases (STDs) such as AIDS.

Barrier methods of contraception

The barrier methods of contraception generally used by teenagers are the male condom, the female condom and spermicides in the form of foam.

The male condom

The male condom is the only method of contraception boys can use. It's really just a rubber tube. It's closed at one end like the finger of a glove so that when a boy puts it over his penis it stops the sperm going inside a girl's body. An advantage of using male condoms is that a boy can take an active part in using contraception. It's not just left to the girl.

There is more information on the AVERT website about using condoms as well as the different types.

The female condom

The female condom is a fairly new barrier method. It is not as widely available as the male condom and it is more expensive. It is however very useful when the man either will not, or cannot, use a male condom.

It's a good idea to try to practise with condoms before having sex. You can get used to touching them, and it might help you feel more confident about using them when you do have sex.

Spermicides

Spermicides are chemical agents that keep sperm from travelling up into the cervix. Spermicide comes in different forms including the sponge, vaginal pessaries which melt in the vagina, and foam which is squirted into the vagina from an aerosol. It is usually spermicide in the form of foam which is used by young people.

Spermicides are not very effective against pregnancy when used on their own, but they can be used at the same time as the male condom which is then very effective. The male condom and spermicide when used together are a good combination for providing effective protection against both pregnancy and STDs such as AIDS.

Some condoms are also available with a spermicide (Nonoxynol 9) added. A spermicidal lubricant also aims to provide an additional level of protection if some semen happens to leak out of the condom. This can help to reduce the likelihood of pregnancy, but regular use of Nonoxynol 9 can cause an allergic reaction in some people, resulting in little sores which can actually make the transmission of HIV more likely. Nonoxynol 9 is a suitable spermicide only for women who are HIV-negative and are at low risk of exposure to HIV or other STIs and only for vaginal sex.

Hormonal methods of contraception

There are two main types of hormonal contraceptive which can be used by teens. If used properly both are extremely effective in providing protection against pregnancy. But they provide no protection at all against sexually-transmitted diseases. For very good protection against both pregnancy and sexually-transmitted diseases such as AIDS, a hormonal method should be used at the same time as the male condom.

The barrier methods of contraception generally used by teenagers are the male condom, the female condom and spermicides in the form of foam

---

The contraceptive pill (sometimes known as the birth control pill)

■ What does 'going on the pill' mean?

People often talk (particularly in the UK) about being 'on the pill'. This means they are using the oral contraceptive pill as a method of contraception. This has nothing to do with oral sex, and just means that the contraceptive is in pill form which the girl swallows.

■ How does it work?

The pill contains chemicals called hormones. One type of pill called the combined pill has two hormones called oestrogen and progestogen. The combined pill stops the release of an egg every month – but doesn't stop periods.

The other type of pill only has progestogen in it. It works by altering the mucous lining of the vagina to make it thicker. The sperm cannot then get through, and as the sperm can't meet the egg, the girl can't get pregnant.

■ What do you do?

Usually the girl has to take one pill every day for about three weeks in every month. It is very important not to forget to take these pills. If this happens, protection against pregnancy is lost. The progestogen-only pill also has to be taken at the same time every day.

■ How effective is the pill?

It is a very effective method of contraception. If the pill is taken exactly according to the instructions, the chance of pregnancy occurring is practically nil. A disadvantage of the pill is that it does not provide any protection against STDs. For very good protection against both pregnancy and STDs, the birth control pill should be used at the same time as the male condom.

Injectable hormonal contraceptive

■ How do you use it? How does it work?

The most popular form of this type of contraception, Depo-Provera, involves the girl having an injection once every 12 weeks. The injection is of the hormone progestogen. The injection works in the same way in the body as the progestogen-only pill, but has the advantage that you do not have to remember to take a pill every day.

It does however have the same disadvantage as the hormonal pill, in that it provides no protection against STDs.

■ The above information is reprinted with kind permission from AVERT. Visit www.avert.org for more information.

© AVERT

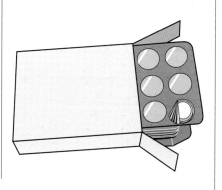

Sexually-transmitted infections

Information from fpa

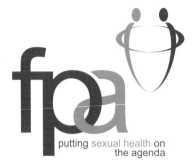

putting sexual health on the agenda

What is a sexually-transmitted infection?

If one person has an infection it can pass to another person through vaginal, anal or oral sex. Infections spread in this way are known as sexually-transmitted infections (STIs). Anyone who has sex can get an STI. You don't need to have lots of sexual partners. Both men and women can get, and pass on, STIs.

Most STIs are easily treated, but treatment should be started as soon as possible. For some infections, such as HIV (the virus that causes AIDS), there is currently no cure and the treatment can be complicated. If left untreated, many STIs can be painful and uncomfortable or, at worst, cause permanent damage to your health and fertility.

How will I know if I have an infection?

Not everyone who has an STI has signs and/or symptoms. Sometimes these don't appear for months and sometimes they go away, but you can still have the infection. If you experience any of the following you should seek advice:

- unusual discharge from the vagina;
- discharge from the penis;
- pain or burning when you pass urine;
- itches, rashes, lumps or blisters around the genitals or anus;
- pain and/or bleeding during sex;
- bleeding between periods (including women who are using hormonal contraception);
- bleeding after sex;
- pain in the testicles or lower abdomen.

Even if you don't have any signs and/or symptoms you may also wish to seek advice or have a check-up, particularly if:

- you have had unprotected sex with a new partner recently;
- you or your sexual partner have sex with other people without using a condom;
- your sexual partner has any symptoms.

Symptoms, however, can vary from infection to infection and many people show no symptoms at all. It is not uncommon to have more than one infection at the same time.

Most STIs can be completely cured if found early enough and may only require you to take a course of antibiotics. However, if left untreated these infections can be painful and uncomfortable or, at worst, cause permanent damage to your health and fertility.

How to avoid sexually-transmitted infections

Using a condom (male or female) correctly and consistently when you have sex will prevent the transmission of most STIs including HIV. However, there are also several things that you can do to make sex safer.

Be prepared

- Discuss with your partner before you have sex how you will both protect yourselves.
- Become familiar with how to use condoms.
- Have a supply of condoms ready (these are free from family planning and sexual health clinics).
- There are lots of choices of condoms so try a different one if you are not happy with the ones you use now.
- Learn about how infections are spread, what symptoms to look for, and where to go for help if you are worried.

Take action

- Have a routine check up at a genitourinary medicine (GUM)/ sexual health clinic (free!).
- If you or your partner have symptoms or think you might have an infection, seek advice before you have any more sex.
- Tell your partner if you have an infection so they can be treated too.

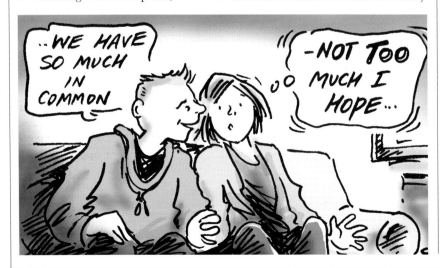

..WE HAVE SO MUCH IN COMMON

-NOT TOO MUCH I HOPE...

Where to go for help and advice

GUM/sexual health clinics specialise in diagnosing and treating all STIs. Most large hospitals have a GUM clinic. You can find details of your nearest clinic by:

- going to the 'I need help' section on the fpa website (www.fpa.org. uk);
- calling fpa's helpline on 0845 310 1334 (Monday to Friday 9.00am-6.00pm);
- looking in the phone book under genitourinary medicine, STD or VD;
- calling the Sexual Health Line on 0800 567 123 (24hrs);
- calling NHS Direct on 0845 46 47 (24hrs).

Facts about GUM/sexual health clinics

- You can refer yourself to any clinic in the country.
- All tests and treatment are free.
- The service is completely confidential.
- Your GP is not informed without your permission.
- People of any age or sexual orientation can attend the clinic.
- If you have an infection then the staff at the clinic can give you help in working out how to tell your current and past partners. This is advised, though it is not compulsory.
- You may need an appointment so ring before you go.

- They can get very busy so be prepared to wait for an appointment and for the first visit to the clinic to take a couple of hours.

If there isn't a clinic near you then you can also get advice from your doctor, your practice nurse or school nurse, a family planning clinic or young people's clinic.

If you would like information about other sexually-transmitted infections you can telephone the fpa helpline on 0845 310 1334 or visit www.ssha.info or www.playingsafely. co.uk.

- The above information is reprinted with kind permission from fpa. Visit www.fpa.org.uk for more information.

© fpa

Young people unaware of sexual health risks

Young people unaware of risks of sexually-transmitted infections and HIV

To mark National Condom Week (8-13 May), the National AIDS Trust is calling for urgent improvements in the education of young people about HIV and other sexually-transmitted infections (STIs) and about the use of condoms.

A quarter of young people aged 15 to 24 years stop using condoms when they or their partner is on the pill

An Ipsos MORI survey, commissioned by the National AIDS Trust, found that a quarter of young people aged 15 to 24 years stop using condoms when they or their partner is on the pill. Yet the pill offers no protection against HIV or STIs. The survey also found that public awareness of how HIV is transmitted has seriously declined over the last five years.

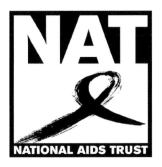

The National AIDS Trust supports the general consensus among professionals that comprehensive sex and relationships education should be a compulsory part of the national curriculum.

Deborah Jack, chief executive of the National AIDS Trust, said:

'Too many young people fail to realise that using a condom with a new sexual partner is a vital protection not only against pregnancy but also against HIV and other sexually-transmitted infections.

'The government must act now to ensure consistent education around condoms and sexual health in schools, ending the current postcode lottery.'

Other findings

- Women are more likely to use condoms than men; 53% of women say they would always use a condom with a new sexual partner, compared to 39% of men.
- 55% of young people would always use a condom with a new sexual partner, compared with 22% who would 'usually' and 12% 'sometimes' use a condom with a new sexual partner.

To see a full copy of the Ipsos MORI report visit www.nat.org.uk.

National Condom Week (8-13 May) is an annual sexual health awareness campaign sponsored by Durex with the support of the National AIDS Trust and other sexual health organisations. For more information about the National Condom Week campaign visit www. hesaysyousay.co.uk.
8 May 2006

- Information from the National AIDS Trust. Visit www.nat.org.uk.
© National AIDS Trust

Wise up: chlamydia

Danielle's story

I found out that I could have an STI a week before my first GCSE. I had been seeing this boy for about a month – he was a couple of years older than me and I really liked him. Things were going really well and we started sleeping together. In the first couple of weeks we used a condom as I definitely didn't want to get pregnant! But then my boyfriend started saying he had heard they could split and he found them awkward. So I decided that I would go on the pill. I had heard a bit about STIs though and knew that condoms helped prevent them so thought that we could use them as well for a bit.

When I told him I was on the pill he was like, 'well what do we want to use condoms for?'

He said sex would be much better without them. The first night we had sex without a condom I'd had a few drinks and I think that made me a bit less bothered about using the condom – plus I thought, well I'm on the pill so I won't get pregnant. Anyway, for about a week everything was great.

Then one night he came round to my house and told me something that totally changed everything.

He had been seeing this girl before me and had slept with her loads of times without using a condom. I knew that he had seen other girls before me but didn't think to ask much about his sex life – I guess I didn't want to know. Anyway, that week his ex-girlfriend had rung him and said she needed to speak to him. When he met her she told him that she had been to the doctors who told her that she had an STI – chlamydia – meaning that he could have it as well. He had already been to the doctors and had it checked out. Turned out that he also had it.

I was confused, I started to panic and then just told my boyfriend I didn't want to see him again.

As soon as he had left I fell on my bed, turned on my music loud and just cried. All that kept going through my head was what people would say. I really thought I'd screwed up my life.

Next morning I went to see my best mate. I felt so stupid and ashamed. I was really worried she would tell other people. It turned out she was really cool and I don't know what I would have done without her. She calmed me down a bit and said we could go to the doctor's together.

The doctor was brilliant. She explained everything clearly and said that whatever happened would be treated confidentially.

She told me that chlamydia was a common STI and often didn't have any symptoms.

However, sometimes you can get a discharge from your vagina, pain going for a wee or during sex, stomach pain and irregular periods. I didn't have any of these things and it worried me that I could have gone on for ages not knowing about the infection.

The doctor also told me that if you don't get it treated early enough it can affect your chances of ever having a baby.

Luckily for me, my boyfriend had warned me and I found out about it early enough. The doctor took a urine sample and told me that she would need to do some tests.

When I went back the results were positive.

I thought I was prepared to hear the worst but I wasn't and I burst into tears. The doctor was great, she talked me through everything and said that it was unlikely there would be any long-term damage. She prescribed the antibiotics for me and told me to come back and see her in a couple of weeks.

Luckily for me everything turned out alright.

The antibiotics worked and the chlamydia cleared. I was also really lucky that I had a fantastic friend and brilliant doctor who both really helped me through it and I suppose

that my boyfriend was honest with me.

If you do find yourself in my situation or even have unprotected sex, I think the main thing is to take some action as quickly as possible. Go and see someone who can help you and from my experience they will be really supportive and kind.

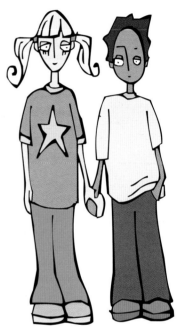

As it is I was lucky, I managed to sort my head out and do my exams.

As for my boyfriend, I avoided him for the first couple of weeks but I did eventually bump into him in town. We did speak about it and it was alright but I couldn't go back to him. He also had the chlamydia sorted out but I just didn't feel the same about him. I don't think it was just his fault though, 'cos I had a choice too.

Now I always use a condom and, though it may be a bit over the top, I wouldn't sleep with a guy without a condom unless he brought along the test results form a doctor to prove that he didn't have an STI.

■ The above information is reprinted with kind permission from RUThinking. Visit www.ruthinking.co.uk for more information.

© RUThinking

Depression in children and young people

Mental health and growing up

What is depression?

Most people, children as well as adults, feel low or 'blue' occasionally. Feeling sad is a normal reaction to experiences that are stressful or upsetting.

When these feelings go on and on, or dominate and interfere with your whole life, it can become an illness. This illness is called 'depression'. Depression probably affects one in every 200 children under 12 years old and two to three in every 100 teenagers.

What are the signs of depression?

- Being moody and irritable – easily upset, 'ratty' or tearful.
- Becoming withdrawn – avoiding friends, family and regular activities.
- Feeling guilty or bad, being self-critical and self-blaming – hating yourself.
- Feeling unhappy, miserable and lonely a lot of the time.

Depression probably affects one in every 200 children under 12 years old and two to three in every 100 teenagers

---

- Feeling hopeless and wanting to die.
- Finding it difficult to concentrate.
- Not looking after your personal appearance.
- Changes in sleep pattern: sleeping too little or too much.
- Tiredness and lack of energy.
- Changes in appetite.
- Frequent minor health problems, such as headaches or stomach-aches.

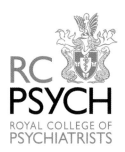

- Some people believe they are ugly, guilty and have done terrible things.

If you have all or most of these signs and have had them over a long period of time, it may mean that you are depressed. You may find it very difficult to talk about how you are feeling.

What causes depression?

Depression is usually caused by a mixture of things, rather than any one thing alone.

Events or personal experiences can be a trigger. These include family breakdown, the death or loss of a loved one, neglect, abuse, bullying and physical illness. Depression can also be triggered if too many changes happen in your life too quickly.

Risk factors

People are more at risk of becoming depressed if they are under a lot of stress, have no one to share their worries with, and lack practical support.

Biological factors

Depression may run in families due to genetic factors. It is also more common in girls and women compared to boys.

Depression seems to be linked with chemical changes in the part of the brain that controls mood. These changes prevent normal functioning of the brain and cause many of the symptoms of depression.

Where can I get help?

There are a lot of things that can be done to help people who suffer from depression.

Helping yourself

Simply talking to someone you trust, and who you feel understands, can lighten the burden. It can also make it easier to work out practical solutions to problems. For example, if you are stressed out by exams, you should talk to your teacher or school counsellor.

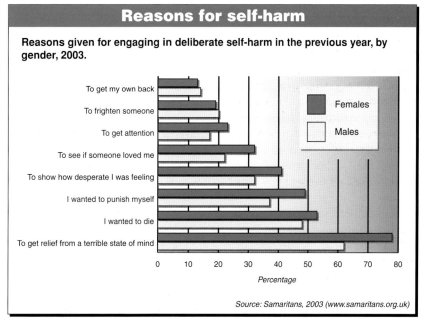

Reasons for self-harm

Reasons given for engaging in deliberate self-harm in the previous year, by gender, 2003.

Source: Samaritans, 2003 (www.samaritans.org.uk)

If you are worried about being pregnant, you should go and see your general practitioner or family planning clinic. Here are some things to remember:

- talk to someone who can help;
- keep as active and occupied as possible, but don't overstress yourself;
- you are not alone – depression is a common problem and can be overcome.

How parents and teachers can help

It can be very hard for young people to put their feelings into words. You can help by asking sympathetically how they are feeling, and listening to them.

When specialist help is needed

If the depression is dragging on and causing serious difficulties, it's important to seek treatment. Your general practitioner will be able to advise you about what help is available and to arrange a referral to the local child and adolescent mental health service.

Many young people will get better on their own with support and understanding. For those whose symptoms are severe and persistent, The National Institute of Clinical Excellence (NICE) recommends that the young person is treated initially with a psychological therapy, such as cognitive behavioural therapy (CBT), for three months. CBT is a type of talking treatment that helps someone understand their thoughts, feelings and behaviour (see Royal College of Psychiatrists leaflet on CBT).

Antidepressant medication should only be used with a psychological therapy such as CBT. Antidepressant medication needs to be taken for six months after the young person feels better. Mild depression should not be treated with antidepressants, but instead with general help and support (see Royal College of Psychiatrists' leaflet on antidepressants).

There is evidence that some antidepressants called SSRIs (Selective Serotonin Re-uptake Inhibitors) can increase thoughts of suicide. For this age group, fluoxetine, which is an SSRI antidepressant, can be used and research has shown that the benefits outweigh the risks. None of the antidepressants are licensed for use in young people under the age of 18 and should only be used by child and adolescent psychiatrists, after a careful assessment. Weekly monitoring of how the young person is feeling will happen in the first four weeks, and then regularly after that.

- The above information is reprinted with kind permission from the Royal College of Psychiatrists. For more information on this and other topics, please visit the Royal College of Psychiatrists' website at www.rcpsych.ac.uk.

© Royal College of Psychiatrists

Not just skin deep

Acne's not just a skin condition; it can toy with your emotions too

Your face is the first thing that people notice when they see you. If you've got a spot on your face, it's difficult not to feel conscious that whoever you're speaking to is gawping right at the offending blemish.

Having one spot is bad enough, but a recent survey says that around 25 per cent of young people either have or have had the skin condition acne.

Acne is not just a few pimples that pop up every now and again. It can be a distressing and painful long-term condition that not only affects sufferers physically, but mentally and socially too.

The effects of acne vary greatly between sufferers. Some people get it mildly, whereas others suffer from red, angry outbreaks, which can make it seem as if the skin is burning up, with 53 per cent of sufferers claiming the spots are painful.

It's not just your face that can be affected. Acne can also appear on the chest, upper back and shoulders.

Acne can carry on into adulthood, and the longer you have acne, the more likely it is to scar.

It's a common myth that acne is a result of poor personal hygiene or inadequate diet. In fact, acne can be genetic. If you've got acne, the chances are at least one of your parents suffered from it too. Hormone fluctuations and stress can also be responsible for outbreaks.

As if having acne wasn't enough to deal with, sufferers also have a hard time when they're teased by others. In the survey, 28 per cent of young people with acne said that they had been the victim of hurtful comments.

Luckily, acne isn't incurable, and there are a growing number of treatments around that could help. Ask a chemist or your GP for any advice. You may think it's strange to go to the doctor about spots, but it's not just your physical well-being that can be affected by acne, it can be a drain on you emotionally as well.

Most GPs will be understanding and will be able to work out what sort of treatment is best for you. There are many over-the-counter treatments available too, and your pharmacist should be able to recommend something to reduce outbreaks.

Schwarz Pharma, the company who commissioned the survey and provided us with the above statistics, have produced a booklet called 'Don't Suffer – Deal With It!', which offers advice on what to do if you are suffering from acne and gives details about the range of treatments available.

For your free copy, send a stamped addressed A5 envelope to: 'Don't Suffer – Deal With It!', Schwarz Pharma Limited, Schwarz House, East Street, Chesham, Bucks, HP5 1DG.

- The above information is reprinted with kind permission from Need2Know. Visit www.need2know.co.uk for more information.

© Crown copyright

Exam stress

Samaritans advice for students and parents too!

Waiting for exam results is a unique kind of stress for students and parents or guardians, so Samaritans have some advice to make it just a bit more bearable.

Getting the results can be every bit as hard for some students. Samaritans believe they have some practical advice for you on some special information pages to be found at www.samaritans.org/talk/exams/results.shtm.

Panic, anxiety, fear about the future, guilt, despair – these are just some of the feelings students might be going through.

Anyone coping with this stressful time needs a great deal of emotional support, but asking for help is not always easy. Without anyone to confide in, stress, anxiety and fear can be unbearable.

> ### Anyone coping with this stressful time needs a great deal of emotional support, but asking for help is not always easy

High expectations from parents, teachers or friends can push students to the brink, particularly when they feel their results don't quite meet those expectations. Learning how to recognise when they're under stress is one of the first steps towards dealing with it.

If anyone would like to talk in confidence to a trained Samaritan, contact us.

The signs of exam stress

Do you have any of these physical symptoms?

- Lack of sleep.
- Loss of appetite or irregular eating.
- Panic attacks and difficulty breathing.

SAMARITANS

- Tight, knotty feelings in your stomach.
- Low energy and lack of concentration.
- Loss of interest in things around you.

'Karen' explains how stressed she felt while waiting for her exam results:

'I wasn't speaking to my parents, I had all these powerful emotions inside of me that I couldn't bring myself to talk to my friends about. I felt like I was being destroyed by what was going on inside of me. I was just at the end of my line. I didn't know where to go, what to do, I thought I'd gone insane, I just wanted some peace. The only way I thought I could get it was by topping myself. I was totally messed up, out of control. If I hadn't rung Samaritans and got help I think I might have done the most stupid thing that anyone could ever do.'

So, what can you do about it?

- Talk to someone you trust, whether that is a friend, teacher or relative.

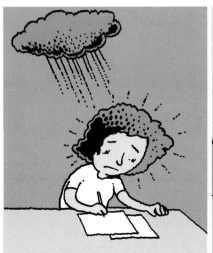

- Eat healthy food regularly.
- Get exercise – walking, running, dancing, sport.
- Get a reasonable amount of sleep.

Why does talking help?

Talking openly about how you really feel can be like opening a door. Talking puts you back in control and reveals the choices you have. Many people feel pressured into hiding their feelings out of embarrassment or concern not to burden family or friends. But hiding under a calm exterior only saves the problem for later and stress can build up until it becomes unbearable. Don't leave it that long. Remember your emotional health is your responsibility and Samaritans is there to help whatever time of the day or night.

'Gary' describes how talking to a Samaritans volunteer helped him:

'I'd like to say how great Samaritans are. I recently phoned them and the bloke I talked to was really calm and friendly.

'He gave me the time that I needed to say difficult things and he called me back so that the call wouldn't appear on the itemised phone bill. No-one there could magically make my life better and totally happy, but talking really did help.

'People reading this who are depressed might not believe that; I know because I was the same. But

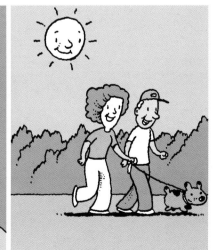

I'd like to say, give it a try – it can't make things worse can it? I also know that there will always be someone at the end of the phone.'

You can call a Samaritan 24 hours a day on 08457 909090 (UK) or 1850 609090 (Republic of Ireland) to talk through stress, depression or anxiety, in total confidence. You can also email us at jo@samaritans. org. If you know someone in distress, encouraging them to phone or email Samaritans will help them take their first step.

Advice for parents

Looking out for the signs of stress

As a parent, of course you want your child to do well in their exams and get brilliant results. But you also, of course, want them to get through the experience. Very few people take their own lives because of their exam results, but for some the stress experienced can seem difficult to cope with.

So, what can you do to make sure that your child is coping?

Begin by keeping a careful eye out for specific signs of stress – these are typical:

- physical symptoms, such as sleeping or eating more or less than usual;
- mental symptoms, such as loss of concentration and interest;
- emotional symptoms such as tears, tantrums, panic attacks;
- addictive symptoms, such as excessive drinking or smoking;
- self-deprecating comments 'I know I'll never pass...' 'John's much brighter than me...';
- calls for help such as 'hanging round', seeming to want to talk. Any one of these signs of stress

should alert you that there's a problem – several signs and alarm bells should be ringing. And be aware that it's not just the hard workers and high achievers who get stressed out. Students with a more moderate track record may be the ones who get most upset because they want to achieve and fear they can't.

Essentially, what children need to know is that they are accepted and valued for their efforts as much as for their achievements, for whether they try rather than whether they succeed

---

Once you suspect that your child is stressed, you'll obviously want to do all you can to reduce that stress. Practical support – like making sure they eat well, sleep enough, and get some exercise – may be difficult to enforce but will make a difference.

Emotional support too is vital. If a young person seems upset or snappy, don't necessarily rush in to calm them down – and so give the impression that they are wrong to feel what they are feeling. The best thing by far is simply to listen – to allow and encourage them to express their worries and fears. Don't feel you have to offer advice or guidance – what they most need, and what will be of most help, is simply space – to talk, to cry, or simply to sit quietly and be.

There may come a point, though, when what a young person needs is one step on from the family support you're offering. Samaritans are always there to offer support and can be contacted at any time of the day or night.

The final and crucial thing to remember, however, is that your attitude will dictate your child's emotions. If you panic, blame or otherwise pressure, then your child's stress will be all the greater. Because, essentially, what children need to know is that they are accepted and valued for their efforts as much as for their achievements, for whether they try rather than whether they succeed. That way they can start to accept themselves, feel good about themselves – and then mysteriously the stress they are under will begin to drop away. (And long term, they will almost certainly succeed more in the future!)

In short, the best message you can give your children is: 'If you've done your best, that's all I can ask. Whatever your results are, I'll still love you.'

Susan Quilliam, agony aunt, FHM.
Based on What To Do When You Really Want To Help But Don't Know How, *by Susan Quilliam, published by Transformation Press. Copies available by ringing Vine House Distribution on 01825 723398, email: sales@vinehouseuk.co.uk or fax: 01825 724188.*

- The above information is reprinted with kind permission from the Samaritans. For more information on this and other topics, please visit their website at www.samaritans.org. uk.

© *Samaritans*

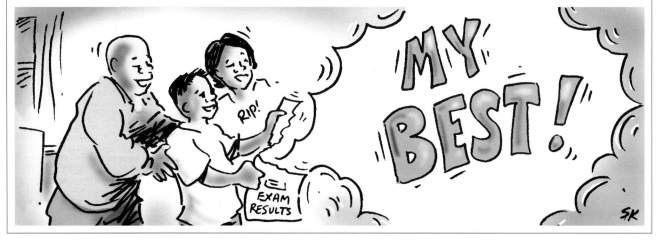

Obesity amongst young people

Information from the National Youth Agency

Obesity and health

Recent research indicating that 11 to 16-year-olds in the UK eat on average 133 pre-packaged ready meals and takeaways a year (nearly three every week) can only be interpreted as bad news. The World Health Organization (WHO) is calling for a limit on the consumption of saturated fats, sugar and salt, especially in snacks, processed foods and drinks, often the prime offenders. At the same time, the World Sugar Research Organisation is lobbying hard against this advice and the US government has said it intends to ignore the recommendations.

Clinicians have referred to rising obesity levels among young people as a 'ticking time-bomb', with one American obesity expert even predicting that parents will outlive their overweight children. Health outcomes for young people who overeat or are overweight are bleak; they will suffer a wide range of chronic diseases ranging from mild ailments such as breathlessness and varicose veins at one extreme to serious conditions such as diabetes and cancer at the other. BBC research reveals that the average young person in Britain spends less time in an average day engaged in physical activity than the average pensioner.

In spite of these ominous signs, there is much good work being delivered to young people concerning their diet and fitness, and this is being administered at all levels – from government at national level to individual youth workers at local level.

National initiatives

- Breakfast clubs: school breakfast clubs are a form of before-school provision serving healthy breakfasts to children who arrive

The National Youth Agency

early. It is reckoned that up to 25 per cent of young people do not currently eat an adequate breakfast.
- 'Five a Day' campaign: fronted by the Department for Education and Skills (DfES), this campaign works with schools to encourage young people to eat at least five portions of fruit and vegetables every day, and to understand the importance of a healthy diet.
- The Growing Schools initiative: the Department for Environment, Food and Rural Affairs (DEFRA) is on the steering group of the Growing Schools initiative which aims to link schools more closely with farming and the countryside in general.
- National Healthy Schools Programme: in 1998, the Department of Health and the Department of Education set up a Healthy Schools Programme in a bid to create a National Healthy Schools Standard (NHSS). The target is that by 2006 all schools with 20 per cent or more free school meal eligibility will become 'Healthy Schools'.

In addition to these government-sponsored schemes, there are numerous ventures at local and regional level designed to foster ideas of healthy lifestyles and healthy eating amongst the young. Centrepoint's food action research and development project, and Shelter's 'Cook It' venture are two such examples.

Young people are bombarded with mixed messages, from the media, from their peers, from family and other sources. Good practice with young people is likely to result

from projects that take advantage of joined-up thinking, projects in which all involved can collaborate successfully and work towards a healthier future for individuals and society.

The website www.eatwell.gov.uk for young people is run by the Food Standards Agency and offers up-to-date information on healthy eating, health issues, food labelling and keeping food safe.

Worried about your weight?

The Royal College of Psychiatrists produces a useful series of leaflets called 'Mental Health and Growing Up'. The aim of these leaflets is to provide practical, up-to-date information about mental health problems (emotional, behavioural and psychiatric disorders) that can affect children and young people.

'Worries about Weight' looks at some of the reasons why people worry about their weight, and offers advice about how to maintain a normal and healthy weight and not let these worries get out of control.

- The above information is reprinted with kind permission from the National Youth Agency. Visit www.youthinformation.com for more information.

© *National Youth Agency*

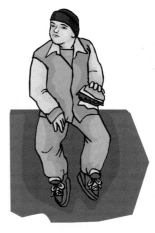

Burger boy and sporty girl

Children and young people's attitudes towards food in school

Key findings from interviews with children and young people

- Children and young people have very strongly developed ideas about health and obesity which are based on gender and income-related stereotypes often portrayed in the media.

- These stereotypes have a strong influence on children's food choices as they do not want to differ from their peers.

- Taste and money play a significant part in what children and young people choose to eat and fast food is viewed as the most tasty and desirable food.

The more choice children and young people have, the less likely they are to eat a healthy, nutritionally-balanced meal

---

- In the context of school, peer pressure strongly influences children's food choices. Teachers, on the other hand, are believed to have no influence on food preferences.

- There is an expectation among both children and adults that children are supposed to prefer unhealthy food.

- There is a strong link between children's perceptions of the food people eat and their affluence, and especially between the brands children eat and what their family can afford.

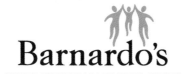

Barnardo's

GIVING CHILDREN BACK THEIR FUTURE

- The contents of lunch boxes are dictated by rigid rules enforced through subtle peer pressure, resulting in lunch boxes that are high in fat, salt and sugar.

- The more choice children and young people have, the less likely they are to eat a healthy, nutritionally-balanced meal. For primary schoolchildren, the limited and repetitive nature of school meals meant that they preferred packed lunches, because they give choice and control. Secondary school lunches offer more choice, but most choices were less healthy with pupils reporting that popular food runs out quickly in the school canteen.

- Very few children are subject to family rules in the home concerning food, with most children believing they are allowed to eat more or less what they like by their parents. This does not vary significantly between primary and secondary schoolchildren.

- Food advertising is influential in persuading children and young people to want and to try the advertised product.

- The obesity-causing environment has infiltrated schools, especially secondary schools, through vending machines and the promotion of energy-dense foods.

- The above information is an extract from the Barnardo's report *Burger Boy and Sporty Girl – children and young people's attitudes towards food in school*, and is reprinted with permission. Visit www.barnardos.uk for more information.

© *Barnardo's*

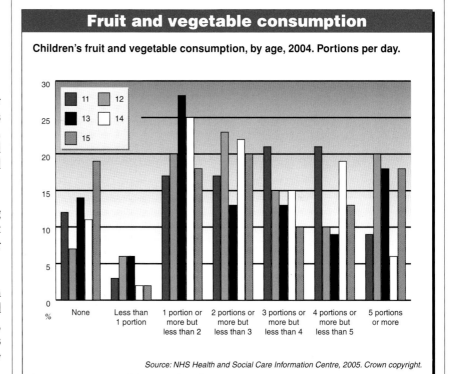

Fruit and vegetable consumption

Children's fruit and vegetable consumption, by age, 2004. Portions per day.

Source: NHS Health and Social Care Information Centre, 2005. Crown copyright.

Food for thought

Information from *0-19*, published by Reed Business Information

With the frenzy surrounding *Jamie's School Dinners* and the subsequent preoccupation with young people's weight and fast-food habits, it seems we have all become obsessed with childhood obesity. But while obesity is an undeniable problem, eating disorders such as anorexia nervosa, bulimia, compulsive eating and selective food refusal continue to blight other children's lives.

According to Hubert Lacey, Professor of Psychiatry at the University of London and director of the St George's Eating Disorders Service, society is rightly concerned about children who are overweight and 'tends to ignore the dangers of slimming'.

While obesity is an undeniable problem, eating disorders such as anorexia nervosa, bulimia, compulsive eating and selective food refusal continue to blight other children's lives

Yet those dangers are worryingly widespread. The Eating Disorders Association estimates the combined total of people diagnosed and undiagnosed with an eating disorder in the UK is around 1.15 million.

Anorexia and bulimia are most common among girls and are closely associated with puberty. As the average age of puberty drops, so does that of children suffering from eating disorders.

Research conducted by ChildLine in 2002 found that three-quarters of calls to the helpline about eating disorders came from children aged between 13 and 16, with some younger children also reporting concerns about their weight. A study

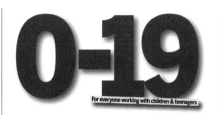

by the *British Journal of Developmental Psychology*, which interviewed 80 children aged between five and eight, found that 47% wanted to be slimmer, with most believing this would make them more popular.

The causes of an eating disorder are seldom simple. Ubiquitous images of skinny, glamorous models may give the impression that thin equals happy, but media influence is only part of the story. Low self-esteem is a common factor, as is stress caused by family problems, bullying and peer pressure. Taking control of food consumption can be a kind of coping mechanism – an attempt to gain control which spirals into a serious problem. Abuse can also be a cause. 'In these cases, the child will wish to disappear, to slip away from view rather than being the controller,' explains Steve Bloomfield, Director of Communications at the Ellern

Mede Centre, which treats eight to 17-year-olds with eating disorders.

Nor is it only girls who are affected. One in 10 sufferers is male and this figure may be rising, perhaps due again to the increasing number of 'perfect' male bodies in the media. Boys are more likely to develop a problem in their later teens and anorexia is difficult to diagnose: over-exercising and developing muscle is more common among boys, making them look fit and meaning it takes longer for the body to look conventionally anorexic. Boys are also less likely to go to the doctor.

Eating disorders can have a destructive impact on family and friends – the sufferer's natural support network. But, according to Bloomfield, recovery comes through communication, which is closely associated with confidentiality.

'It's always advisable to go to the GP,' Broomfield says, 'but a child might fear their doctor is also that of their parents. School nurses and practice nurses therefore play an important role.'

Helplines, text and email support services are available, and some self-help groups operate nationwide. Many

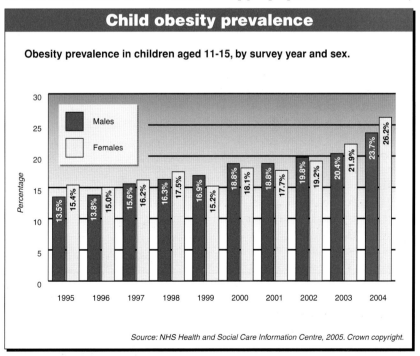

Child obesity prevalence

Obesity prevalence in children aged 11-15, by survey year and sex.

Source: NHS Health and Social Care Information Centre, 2005. Crown copyright.

sufferers require more professional help, though, and Lacey suggests that family-based treatments, particularly in outpatients, have been shown to be effective. However, he adds that patients at low weight often require inpatient treatment. Unfortunately, though, the availability of treatment on the NHS varies widely across the country.

The Eating Disorders Association estimates the combined total of people diagnosed and undiagnosed with an eating disorder in the UK is around 1.15 million

Nor are there any quick fixes. Recovery time is between five and six years, though it can be longer. The disorder can also recur, if triggered by great stress later in life, such as divorce or bereavement. There are similarities to addictions in this regard – sufferers may never be 'cured' but they can recover. Of those children who do not receive treatment, one in five will die prematurely. Those who get help should recover to live a normal life.

'It's not about vanity – it's a form of control'

Gemma Oaten developed an eating disorder aged 11. Now 21, and after a long struggle, she is positive about recovery.

'I never worried about my weight when I was younger. I'd been close friends with the lads at school. But then suddenly they were looking at me differently and there was jealousy from girls. I was a high achiever and people would pick on me – calling me a slag.

'I couldn't control people's opinions but I could control my food. I felt under pressure to achieve and it was a way to escape. When my periods stopped it felt like I was a child again and that's what I wanted... Anorexia crept up on me.

'When I first went to the doctor's they said, "You're not underweight enough yet for it to be a problem." But you don't have to be thin to have an eating disorder. So I decided to make sure I lost enough to get help.

'Anorexia takes over everything. I went to an adolescent unit, but it treated people with all sorts of different problems. They didn't have a clue how to help so my parents took me out of there.

'At 15 I got back to a normal weight but still felt uncomfortable. I got a stomach bug and around that time I became bulimic. It gave me a sense of release from my anger. I was in and out of hospital with low potassium and fainting. It was frightening.

'I'm doing well now. I have difficult times but I have the power not to let it beat me. I can't imagine how I would have managed without my fantastic family. They've had to fight to get me help – it's such a battle and you need funding.

'I see a psychotherapist regularly and that's a big factor. I finally have some consistency – I trust her and she's there for me. But there's still so many who aren't getting help. It's not about vanity, it's nothing to do with that. It's a form of control.'

Warning signs

- A preoccupation with calories and fat grams.
- Frequent weighing.
- Food rituals (eating foods in sequence, not letting certain foods touch each other; cutting food up very small).
- Avoiding eating in public.
- A preoccupation with food.
- Excessive exercise.
- Disappearing to the bathroom after a meal.
- Evidence of use of laxatives, diuretics or vomiting.
- Wearing baggy clothes.
- Irregular or no periods.
- A distorted perception of their own appearance and body weight.

What can help

- Accepting that change must come from the young person and cannot be forced.
- Anticipating some level of denial – eating disorders can be comparable to addictions in this regard.
- Giving the young person a chance to talk and explain their point of view.
- Encouraging the young person to seek professional help.
- Being consistent; parents especially should try to agree on a strategy and stick to it.

What does not help

- Offering bribes or rewards to make the child change eating behaviours.
- Making threats and being confrontational.
- Ignoring the problem in the hope it will go away without help.

1 December 2005

- Information from *0-19*, published by Reed Business Information. Visit www.0-19.co.uk for more.

© *Reed Business Information*

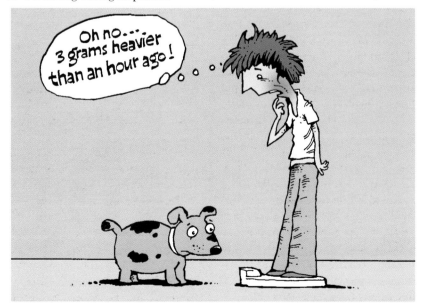

Children and suicide

Sharp rise in suicide calls, warns ChildLine

Worrying numbers of the UK's young people are considering taking their own lives in a desperate attempt to escape their problems. That's the warning from ChildLine – now part of the NSPCC – which today (15 March 2006) reveals an alarming 14% rise in calls from suicidal children to its free, 24-hour helpline.

ChildLine is calling on the Department of Health, the Scottish Executive and the Welsh Assembly Government to undertake an in-depth study of young suicides and suicide attempts, including talking to children who have attempted suicide, to help ensure that children on the verge of suicide get prompt access to the help they so desperately need.

In addition, ChildLine believes that every school should have a senior staff member responsible for safeguarding and promoting the welfare of pupils and ensuring that their mental health and well-being needs are met. This must be backed up by provision of on-site counselling services and other support structures, including schemes that enable children to learn to help and support each other.

ChildLine supporter and TV psychologist Dr Tanya Byron is backing the campaign. She says: 'Suicide is a tragedy, which can and must be prevented. Last year 1,039 children and young people spoke to ChildLine about feeling suicidal. When children and young people have thoughts of suicide, they rarely come out of the blue. Often children will talk about multiple problems – which can include physical or sexual abuse, neglect, stress and low self-esteem – which have led them to this absolute crisis point. It's vital that young people know they don't have to suffer in silence. I would urge children and young people who are feeling suicidal – or who have any other problems – to call ChildLine free at any time on 0800 1111.'

Why do young people feel suicidal?

ChildLine's counsellors know there are no simple explanations for suicidal behaviour – and therefore no quick-fix solutions. Calls to ChildLine show that abuse, constant rows with someone close, bullying, stress over exams, and worries about the future are just some of the things that can cause feelings of anxiety, low self-esteem, hopelessness and isolation in some young people. Groups particularly at risk of suicide include unemployed or homeless young people, young gay men and women, and young people who have problems with drugs.

Young people tell ChildLine how important it is for them to have someone who will take the time to listen and be there for them at a time of crisis. Just picking up the phone to ChildLine is an important step for them to take, because being taken seriously by an adult can make all the difference between a young person choosing to live or die.

Tragically, some young people who talk to ChildLine about feeling suicidal have actually made an attempt – such as an overdose – just before calling, and need immediate medical help.

President of ChildLine, Esther Rantzen, says: 'All young death is agonising but suicide is among the cruellest of all – because it's preventable. One child rang Child-Line from her science lesson; she had already taken an overdose. Another teenage couple had taken a suicide pact and rang having cut their wrists. For these children, ChildLine was literally a lifeline – those lives were saved. But just imagine if those children had not been able to get through to ChildLine? Of the 4,500 children who try to get through to ChildLine each day, nearly half will not get through because there are not enough funds to answer them.'

This year ChildLine joined with the NSPCC and has set a target of 20 million pounds to answer thousands more children during the helpline's 20th birthday year. To help Child-Line to be there for every child in need and support the 20th Birthday Appeal, call 0800 876 6000.

Notes

1. Last year (1 April 2004-31 March 2005) 1,039 children and young people called ChildLine primarily about feeling suicidal. This represents an increase of 14% compared to 910 children calling primarily about suicide during the year 2003-2004.
2. An additional 1,698 children calling ChildLine last year (1 April 2004-31 March 2005) mentioned suicide in relation to other problems.
3. Where counsellors were able to establish the age of the caller, 42% of the calls regarding suicide were from 16 to 18-year-olds. Normally only 18% of calls to ChildLine are from this older age bracket.
4. The girl to boy ratio for suicide as a main problem in children's calls is currently 5:1 – the ratio for all calls is 3:1. This reflects the fact that more girls than boys try to commit suicide (statistics from MIND).

15 March 2006

■ The above information is re-printed with kind permission from ChildLine. Visit www.childline.org.uk for more information. ChildLine and the NSPCC joining together for children.

© NSPCC

Self-harm

Information taken from a ChildLine information sheet

'I can't stop cutting myself. I don't feel alive any more. People pick on me and nobody talks to me – I feel like I'm invisible.' Linzi, 15

What is self-harm?

Self-harm is when people set out to harm themselves deliberately, sometimes in a hidden way. Self-harm can include cutting, burning, bruising or poisoning, but does not usually mean that someone wants to commit suicide.

But, if people are not helped to stop self-harming, there is a risk that their urge to hurt themselves could grow into a stronger wish to end their lives.

The number of children talking to ChildLine's counsellors about self-harm has grown steadily over the last 10 years. Over 60 per cent of the young people who call us about self-harm are aged between 12 and 15, and 12 times as many girls call about self-harming as boys.

Cutting is the most common form of self-harm that ChildLine hears about, but callers also talk about harming their bodies in other ways, such as deliberately bruising themselves, banging their heads against walls, pulling out their hair, burning themselves, falling over, or breaking an arm or leg.

How does ChildLine help?

ChildLine's counsellors know that there is a difference between self-harming and wanting to commit suicide. But, when some young people call to talk about self-harm, they may need immediate medical attention. The counsellors listen carefully to each caller's situation at that moment and decide if medical help is needed.

Self-harm can include cutting, burning, bruising or poisoning, but does not usually mean that someone wants to commit suicide

---

Young people who call feel that it is important that ChildLine is confidential. They know that ChildLine is a safe place for them to talk about their feelings – they will not be judged, blamed or criticised.

Although callers to ChildLine need help, they do not want people to know that they self-harm or to be forced to tell their family before they are ready. For some, the ChildLine counsellor is the first person they tell about their self-harm, but many others have already told someone before.

ChildLine counsellors talk to young people about how and when they hurt themselves, to try to find out how they feel before, during and after. This may help to find out why they are self-harming or what starts it

---

Self-harm and suicide

An overview

- Self-harm encompasses a wide variety of behaviours and acts – different terms such as attempted suicide or parasuicide may also be used to describe it. These acts involve differing degrees of risk to life, and differing degrees of suicidal intent, but all speak of intense emotional distress in the person who deliberately harms themselves.
- People who have self-harmed are at greatly-increased risk of suicide and should have access to assessment and support.
- The UK has one of the highest rates of self-harm in Europe, at 400 per 100,000 population. It is estimated that there are at least 170,000 cases of self-harm which come to hospital attention each year. Many more incidents of self-harming behaviour probably take place but are not included in any statistics because people may choose not to seek medical help.
- In the Republic of Ireland, the rate is estimated at 196 per 100,000 population. Over 10,000 cases of parasuicide are seen in Irish hospitals every year.
- The group with the highest rates of self-harm are young women aged 15 to 19 years. In all age groups, females are more likely to self-harm than males.
- Young males, however, show the most alarming increases in rates of self-harm.
- By far the most common method of self-harm which comes to hospital attention is overdose of drugs, most often paracetamol. Reduction in pack sizes of paracetamol sold over the counter in the UK has resulted in reduced self-harm.
- In recognition of the seriousness of self-harm, the associated risk of suicide and the considerable distress it causes to individuals and those around them, national strategies have been developed by English, Scottish and Irish government departments within the last three years.

March 2005

- The above information is an extract from information provided by the Samaritans entitled 'Self-harm and Suicide' and is reprinted with permission. Visit www.samaritans.org.uk to view the full text and references.

© Samaritans

off, such as bullying, abuse or family tensions. ChildLine helps callers to find ways to stop self-harming – ways that they themselves are able to follow, or else they continue to find it difficult to stop hurting themselves.

ChildLine also suggests that callers ring again the next time they feel like self-harming. Unlike many other services, ChildLine is easy to reach and offers comfort, advice and protection 24 hours a day.

Why do children and young people self-harm?

'I cut myself when I'm angry. It hurts but it helps my anger.' Lisa, 11

Young people who speak to ChildLine about self-harm talk about their anger and frustration at things that are going on in their lives and the strong emotions that they need to release.

Callers tell ChildLine that the self-harm removes the other pain they feel, and they feel exhilarated while it is happening. But some say they feel guilty afterwards. This guilt may stop some young people from seeking help, or from telling a parent or carer, because they do not want anyone to think they were trying to commit suicide.

Lily said she had been cutting her arms and legs for about five months:

'It feels good when I'm doing it, but then it hurts.'

Lily cut herself two to three times a week whenever something happened. She told the school nurse and saw a counsellor once, but then had trouble setting up another appointment.

Often the self-harm seems to have started because of a crisis or ongoing difficulty in young callers' lives, such as sexual abuse (either ongoing or in the past), divorce, going into care, or the death of someone close.

Chrissie's parents were arguing all the time and making her so anxious she kept cutting her arms and legs:

'I don't think they love me. They argue all the time and my dad sometimes hits out at me.'

Emma, 14, asked ChildLine to help her stop cutting herself and beating herself up. Her best friend

had died in a car crash a year ago, and now she was worried about exams in school.

In particular, many of the young people tell counsellors that their self-harm is linked to sexual abuse they have suffered. These tend to be older teenagers, who talk about being depressed and hating themselves and their bodies because of what happened to them. A number of these callers talk about having flashbacks to the abuse, and the cutting takes away these memories.

Shell, 14, said:

'I cut myself when I feel sad, upset and alone.'

A 15-year-old girl called because her brother had been sexually abusing her for 18 months and she knew it was not right. She said she self-harms to punish herself.

As with other problems, such as eating disorders, depression, and substance abuse, young people who call ChildLine for help with self-harm mainly talk about a loss of control over their lives. By inflicting injury and pain on their bodies, these callers seem to regain a sense of control and personal ownership of their lives.

Who should I tell about self-harming?

'I told my teacher, but still couldn't stop doing it.' Macie, 14

Children and young people calling about self-harm often say it is hard to stop and want to understand why they do this to themselves. Before contacting ChildLine, nearly half the callers had already told someone (such as a friend, parent, teacher, counsellor or doctor) about the problem.

But many young people do not want to tell anyone, either because they are worried about the shame, or because people will think they are mad or cannot be cured.

Young people calling about self-harm are more likely to speak to their friends than anyone else. Friends are supportive, do not judge and care deeply if someone they like is in trouble.

Thousands of young people call ChildLine every year because they are worried about someone they

know. Because of this, ChildLine set up ChildLine in Partnership with Schools (CHIPS), which encourages schoolchildren to help and support each other. This support is good for dealing with problems related to school, such as bullying or exam stress, both of which are reasons given for self-harm by young people.

If you self-harm, you are not alone. Many young people cut, bruise or hurt themselves to cope with stressful and difficult feelings or circumstances.

Between 2002 and 2003 Child-Line heard from over 3,000 children and young people who said they were self-harming or had harmed themselves in the past.

How can I stop self-harming?

One 13-year-old girl told ChildLine that she uses breathing as a way to stop cutting herself:

'I used to cut myself, but now I try to breathe instead to calm down.'

Although it may not be possible to make the causes of self-harm disappear, there are other ways to express strong emotions and to relieve the pain, such as:

- writing down negative feelings on a piece of paper and ripping it up;
- keeping a journal or diary of feelings;
- doing something physical like running or skating, or making a lot of noise;
- calling up a friend and talking, but not necessarily about self-harm.

ChildLine offers children and young people calling about self-harm the chance to talk in confidence about what is happening in their lives. ChildLine is free and available 24 hours a day, 365 days a year. ChildLine counsellors do not blame or criticise callers, but help them to work out how they can stop their self-harming and suggest where they can go for further support or advice.

- The above information is reprinted with kind permission from ChildLine. Visit www.childline.org.uk for more information. ChildLine and the NSPCC joining together for children.

© NSPCC

Truth hurts

National Inquiry into Self-Harm calls for better responses to young people

The National Inquiry today called on the government to launch a UK-wide initiative to develop better and more appropriate responses to young people who self-harm, starting with an awareness campaign targeted at professionals, parents and young people.

According to the Truth Hurts report, professionals and adults often react inappropriately to disclosure of self-harm, which frequently makes the situation worse

---

The recommendation is made in *Truth Hurts*, the final report by the National Inquiry into Self-Harm, which reveals that young people who self-harm are more likely to turn to friends their own age for help, rather than relatives, teachers or GPs. Widespread misunderstandings about self-harm among professionals and relatives are preventing young people who self-harm from seeking and getting support. Yet little information is available to help parents and professionals learn to deal with self-harm effectively.

According to the *Truth Hurts* report, professionals and adults often react inappropriately to disclosure of self-harm, which frequently makes the situation worse. There is a tendency for adults to focus solely on the self-harming behaviour rather than the underlying causes. Young people often hurt themselves for long periods of time without ever disclosing their self-harm.

The two-year Inquiry, jointly run by the Camelot Foundation and the Mental Health Foundation, has found that health, education and social care professionals are not

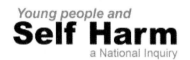

Young people and Self Harm a National Inquiry

receiving the guidance or formal training they need to support young people who self-harm. Nor do professionals feel they receive sufficient personal support to deal with self-harm cases. The Inquiry reveals that education professionals would like information and advice about self-harm to be provided in all schools across the UK.

The Inquiry has learned that a number of circumstances can lead a person to begin self-harming, such as being bullied at school, not getting on with parents, anxiety about academic performance, parental divorce, bereavement, unwanted pregnancy, experience of sexual, physical or emotional abuse in earlier childhood, and difficulties associated with sexuality.

Self-harm is a coping mechanism which enables a person to express difficult emotions. Young people who hurt themselves often feel that physical pain is easier to deal with than the emotional pain they are experiencing, because it is tangible. But the behaviour only provides temporary relief and fails to deal with the underlying issues that a young person is facing.

According to *Truth Hurts*, stopping or reducing self-harming behaviour is a long process. Alternative coping strategies need to be learned to deal with difficult life circumstances and emotions. The Inquiry's research says that young people seeking help would like counselling, drop-in centres and facilitated self-help groups to be made available. The report asserts that schools provide an appropriate setting in which young people would

like to see external individuals and organisations, independent of schools, provide information and advice.

Chair of the Inquiry, Catherine McLoughlin CBE, said; 'It is vital that everyone who comes into contact with young people has a basic understanding of what self-harm is, why people do it, and how to respond appropriately. At the very least they should avoid being judgemental towards young people who disclose self-harm, should treat them with care and respect and should acknowledge the emotional distress they are clearly experiencing.'

Susan Elizabeth, director of the Camelot Foundation, said: 'There is an urgent need to provide information and guidance for parents and carers, friends and professionals – people are struggling in the dark. We must get rid of the fear, misunderstanding and stigma that surrounds self-harm.'

Dr Andrew McCulloch, chief executive of the Mental Health Foundation, said: 'Self-harm is evidently a symptom of mental and emotional distress. We need to look past the behaviour and provide understanding, support and effective services for young people in the UK.'
26 March 2006

■ The above information is reprinted with kind permission from the National Inquiry into Self-Harm. Visit www.selfharmuk.org for more information.
© Camelot Foundation and the Mental Health Foundation

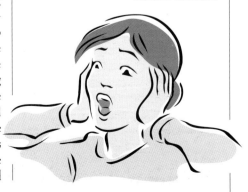

My story

Information on self-harm

'Ok, so my story is pretty simple, I'm an ordinary girl, with an ordinary life. I suppose I had never particularly liked myself, but that wasn't so much of an issue. When I was about 12 everything in my life started to fall apart, I found out that I had a condition called alopecia which meant that my hair fell out. Well, some of it. I was desperate for no one to find out, because we had a uniform at school, I couldn't wear a hat, so I started to get bullied. Nothing awful, but it was the times that I wasn't bullied that were the worst, because I was always waiting.

> **'I knew that I was always a strong one, I couldn't cry, I couldn't get angry, people had to rely on me. So I started to self-harm'**

I shut myself off from the world, I didn't want to feel the pain that they were trying to inflict on me. I knew that I was always a strong one, I couldn't cry, I couldn't get angry, people had to rely on me. So I started to self-harm.

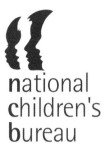

The cycle of self-harm carried on, I didn't want anyone to know, I suppose that I had been an intermittent self-harmer for about three to four years, when my friend found out. We decided together that I needed to tell someone; so I did. I told my teacher. Though I sometimes wish I hadn't, I know if I hadn't got it out in the open I never would have stopped.

Things got worse for a while after I told someone, because I couldn't bear people knowing. But it did get better. I decided that I was worth more that self-harming, that the thing that I was trying to kill inside me wouldn't go away by hurting the outside. I had to tackle that monster in a new way because the old way only hurt him for a second, and each time I hurt he grew stronger.

I had to talk. I know that I will always be a self-harmer, but that doesn't mean I have to hurt myself. I have power within myself to stop, and when I feel like I'm going to break, I ring someone, or I listen to music.

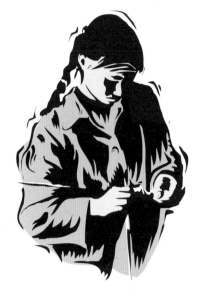

Finally I have found control, not in hurting myself, but in stopping. In finally saying no. Anyone can do it, but if you can't then you are not a failure. Just trust and know, that you will one day find that you are too special to hurt yourself, and most importantly there is a way out. Never accept the lie that self-harm is the only way.'

■ The above information is reprinted with kind permission from the National Children's Bureau (NCB). For more information, please visit the NCB website dedicated to the problem of self-harm at www.selfharmuk.org.uk.

© NCB

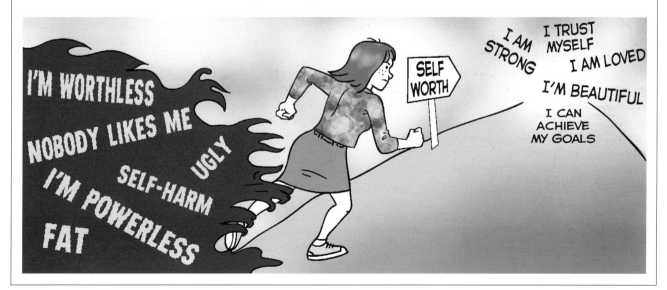

■ 30% of 14 to 15-year-old females and 22% of 14 to 15-year-old males surveyed had nothing at all to eat for breakfast 'this' morning. (page 1)

■ 24% of 14 to 15-year-old females and 14% of 14 to 15-year-old males surveyed smoked at least one cigarette during the previous week. (page 2)

■ 27% of 14 to 15-year-old females surveyed described themselves as 'unfit' or 'very unfit'. (page 2)

■ Teenagers in Britain are largely inactive, with 46% of boys and 69% of girls aged 15 to 18 spending less than the recommended one hour a day participating in activities of moderate intensity. (page 6)

■ An estimated 450 young people take up smoking each day, and as a sign of how addictive smoking can be, research has found that 70 per cent of adult smokers originally started smoking between the ages of 11 and 15 years old. (page 8)

■ More than a million adolescents have wanted to self-harm, and more than 800,000 have done so. Nearly one million young people have felt so miserable that they have considered suicide, with more than one in five 18 to 19-year-old girls admitting to feeling this way. (page 9)

■ Young people look for comfort when they're upset or 'down' faster than any other age group, according to research carried out for Samaritans. But they still have emotional 'secrets' they won't share with even their closest friends. (page 10)

■ Half of smokers under the age of 16 who try to buy cigarettes from shops succeed in doing so. (page 11)

■ Children's vulnerability to taking up smoking after trying just a single cigarette can lie dormant for three years or more, according to a study from Cancer Research UK. (page 13)

■ 1,000 children under the age of 15 are admitted to hospital each year with acute alcohol poisoning. (page 16)

■ 27% of 11 to 15-year-olds have used an illicit drug in the last month. (page 17)

■ Alcohol-related deaths have risen by nearly one-fifth in the last four years. (page 18)

■ Eight out of 10 teenagers lose their virginity when they are drunk, feel pressurised into having sex or are not using contraception, a survey has revealed. (page 19)

■ The age at which the majority of 16 to 19-year-olds today first have sexual intercourse is 16. Almost 30% of young men and almost 26% of young women report having intercourse before their 16th birthday. (page 21)

■ An Ipsos MORI survey, commissioned by the National AIDS Trust, found that a quarter of young people aged 15 to 24 years stop using condoms when they or their partner is on the pill. Yet the pill offers no protection against HIV or STIs. (page 25)

■ The majority of males and females who self-harmed said they did so 'to get relief from a terrible state of mind', according to figures from the Samaritans. (page 27)

■ The effects of acne vary greatly between sufferers. Some people get it mildly, whereas others suffer from red, angry outbreaks, which can make it seem as if the skin is burning up, with 53 per cent of sufferers claiming the spots are painful. (page 28)

■ Research indicates that 11 to 16-year-olds in the UK eat on average 133 pre-packaged ready meals and takeaways a year (nearly three every week). (page 31)

■ Children and young people have very strongly-developed ideas about health and obesity which are based on gender and income-related stereotypes often portrayed in the media. (page 32)

■ The Eating Disorders Association estimates the combined total of people diagnosed and undiagnosed with an eating disorder in the UK is around 1.15 million. (page 33)

■ Last year (1 April 2004-31 March 2005) 1,039 children and young people called ChildLine primarily about feeling suicidal. This represents an increase of 14% compared to 910 children calling primarily about suicide during the year 2003-2004. (page 35)

■ By far the most common method of self-harm which comes to hospital attention is overdose of drugs, most often paracetamol. Reduction in pack sizes of paracetamol sold over the counter in the UK has resulted in reduced self-harm. (page 36)

■ Self-harm is a coping mechanism which enables a person to express difficult emotions. Young people who hurt themselves often feel that physical pain is easier to deal with than the emotional pain they are experiencing, because it is tangible. But the behaviour only provides temporary relief and fails to deal with the underlying issues that a young person is facing. (page 38)

GLOSSARY

Acne
A skin condition consisting mainly of red spots on the face. Around 25% of young people either have or have had acne, according to a survey.

Addiction
Physical or psychological dependence on something, either a substance or an activity. Young people are more likely to experiment with substances that contain physically addictive chemicals, such as alcohol, cigarettes or illegal drugs.

Adolescence
The period in our teenage years during which one becomes an adult, after the onset of puberty.

Binge drinking
Drinking significantly more than the recommended daily intake of alcohol units in one session. There is concern that binge drinking is on the rise among young people in the UK, fuelling anti-social behaviour and health problems. 49% of boys and 48% of girls aged 15 had drunk alcohol in the last week, according to a 2003 government survey.

Chlamydia
Chlamydia is the most commonly-diagnosed sexually transmitted infection, with more than 30,000 cases annually. It affects about 10% of young men and women. If untreated, it can spread to other reproductive organs, causing health problems which could include infertility.

Contraception
Anything which prevents conception (pregnancy). The most common methods of birth control among young people are male condoms: latex sheaths which fit over the penis and prevent pregnancy by acting as a barrier, stopping sperm from reaching an egg during intercourse; and the contraceptive pill (often just called 'the pill') – this is taken daily by the girl and contains hormones which prevent an egg from being fertilised. Unlike condoms, however, this method does not also protect against STIs.

Depression
When feeling sad and 'blue' go on and on, or dominate and interfere with your whole life, it can become an illness – depression. Depression probably affects one in every 200 children under 12 years old and two to three in every 100 teenagers.

Eating disorders
Anorexia nervosa, bulimia nervosa and binge eating disorders are psychological illnesses characterised by a serious disturbance in eating, as well as distress or excessive concern about body shape or weight.

Freshers' flu
An ailment common among new students – like conventional flu, it is a disease of the lungs and upper airways, caused by the flu virus. It is the consequence of a sudden, sustained battering to the immune system.

HIV
Human Immunodeficiency Virus, a very dangerous STI which causes AIDS. Unlike most other STIs, it is incurable, so it is very important to use a barrier method of contraception such as a condom, which will prevent its spread.

Meningitis
An infection of the membranes that cover the brain and spinal cord. After children, young adults are most at risk, and everyone under 25 should receive the meningitis C vaccine. This does not protect against meningitis B, the more common but less dangerous infection.

Puberty
The time in a person's life when they reach sexual maturity, becoming capable of reproduction. The body undergoes changes during this period (pubescence), as it moves into adulthood.

Self-harm
When people deliberately set out to hurt themselves through methods such as cutting, poisoning and burning. It does not generally mean that someone wants to commit suicide, but is usually a form of control. The group with the highest rates of self-harm are young women aged 15 to 19. The UK has one of the highest rates of self-harm in Europe.

Sexually-transmitted infections (STIs)
There are many different types of these, including genital herpes, chlamydia, gonorrhoea and HIV. STIs are transmitted by unprotected intimate sexual contact; a barrier method of contraception such as a male condom will prevent the transmission of most STIs, as well as preventing pregnancy. Hormonal methods of contraception such as the Pill are not effective in preventing the spread of STIs, and should be used alongside a barrier contraceptive for full protection.

INDEX

ADDITIONAL RESOURCES

Other Issues *titles*

If you are interested in researching further the issues raised in *Young People and Health*, you may want to read the following titles in the **Issues** series as they contain additional relevant articles:

- Vol. 127 *Eating Disorders* (ISBN 1 86168 366 9)

- Vol. 125 *Understanding Depression* (ISBN 1 86168 364 2)

- Vol. 117 *Self-Esteem and Body Image* (ISBN 1 86168 350 2)

- Vol. 114 *Drug Abuse* (ISBN 1 86168 347 2)

- Vol. 113 *Fitness and Health* (ISBN 1 86168 346 4)

- Vol. 100 *Stress and Anxiety* (ISBN 1 86168 314 6)

- Vol. 96 *Preventing Sexual Diseases* (ISBN 1 86168 304 9)

- Vol. 93 *Binge Drinking* (ISBN 1 86168 301 4)

- Vol. 86 *Smoking and your Health* (ISBN 1 86168 287 5)

- Vol. 80 *The Cannabis Debate* (ISBN 1 86168 275 1)

- Vol. 77 *Self-inflicted Violence* (ISBN 1 86168 266 2)

For more information about these titles, visit our website at www.independence.co.uk/publicationslist

Useful organisations

You may find the websites of the following organisations useful for further research:

- Action on Smoking and Health: www.ash.org.uk

- AVERT: www.avert.org

- Brook Advisory Centres: www.brook.org.uk

- fpa: www.fpa.org.uk

- NCB: www.selfharmuk.org.uk

- Need2Know: www.need2know.co.uk

- The Royal College of Psychiatrists: www.rcpsych.ac.uk

- RUThinking: www.ruthinking.co.uk

- The Samaritans: www.samaritans.org.uk

- Schools Health Education Unit: www.sheu.org.uk

ACKNOWLEDGEMENTS

The publisher is grateful for permission to reproduce the following material.

While every care has been taken to trace and acknowledge copyright, the publisher tenders its apology for any accidental infringement or where copyright has proved untraceable. The publisher would be pleased to come to a suitable arrangement in any such case with the rightful owner.

Chapter One: Overview

Young people into 2006, © SHEU, *Student health issues*, © Telegraph Group Ltd, London 2006, *Nutrition through life: teenagers*, © British Nutrition Foundation, *Addictions: the basics*, © Crown copyright is reproduced with the permission of Her Majesty's Stationery Office, *Adolescent mental health*, © Reed Business Information, *Drug use, smoking and drinking*, © Crown copyright is reproduced with the permission of Her Majesty's Stationery Office, *Young Brits lose stiff upper lip*, © Samaritans.

Chapter Two: Adolescent Health Issues

Young people and smoking, © Action on Smoking and Health, *Smoking and the 'sleeper effect'*, © Cancer Research UK, *Drugs and alcohol*, © Royal College of Psychiatrists, *Alcohol facts for young people*, © Surgery Door, *Substance misuse*, © Barnardo's, *Wide eyed and legless*, © Reed Business

Information, *What teens really think about sex*, © Guardian Newspapers Ltd 2006, *Teenage sexual activity*, © Brook Advisory Centres, *Birth control and contraception for teenagers*, © AVERT, *Sexually-transmitted infections*, © fpa, *Young people unaware of sexual health risks*, © National AIDS Trust, *Wise up: chlamydia*, © RUThinking, *Depression in children and young people*, © Royal College of Psychiatrists, *Not just skin deep*, © Crown copyright is reproduced with the permission of Her Majesty's Stationery Office, *Exam stress*, © Samaritans, *Obesity amongst young people*, © National Youth Agency, *Burger boy and sporty girl*, © Barnardo's, *Food for thought*, © Reed Business Information, *Children and suicide*, © NSPCC, *Self-harm*, © NSPCC, *Self-harm and suicide*, © Samaritans, *Truth hurts*, © Camelot Foundation and the Mental Health Foundation, *My story*, © NCB.

Photographs and illustrations:

Pages 1, 20: Bev Aisbett; pages 4, 12, 39: Angelo Madrid; pages 7, 24, 30: Simon Kneebone; pages 10, 29, 34: Don Hatcher.

Craig Donnellan
Cambridge
September, 2006